# PRAISE FOR RESILIENT THREADS

*Resilient Threads* is a treasure. Mukta Panda has beautifully captured what it means to be a compassionate physician—one who effortlessly dedicates herself to the well-being of not just patients but also colleagues, students and friends alike. Dr. Panda knows what it means to create a psychologically safe workplace—and why it matters for learning, excellence, and full engagement at work. Readers will pick up countless ideas to transform their own workplaces by adopting the author's generous and curious spirit.

—**Amy C. Edmondson, PhD**, Professor, Harvard Business School, author of *The Fearless Organization* and *Building the Future*.

Dr. Mukta Panda has kept her heart alive in a health care system where people too often lose heart. In her new book, *Resilient Threads*, she shows us how to stay close to painful emotions like anxiety, anger, grief, and burnout so that they become sources of energy to challenge and change institutions. Mukta has modeled for her medical students—and readers of any profession—what it means to be on the journey toward "an undivided life." The work of personal and institutional transformation is far from done, but there is hope that it can happen because we see it in Mukta's stories. I'm grateful to Mukta for having the courage to share how she keeps her heart open despite heartbreak, and is teaching her medical students and residents to do the sar̶ Mukta's clinical specialty, but sh̶ ̶vell.

—**Parker J. Palmer,** ̶ning, *The Courage to Teach, A Hidd* ̶peak

D1511062

A powerful, inspiring example of a female physician and mother whose empathy, compassion, and self-care reveal what is needed to get through medical training and revive the good doctor you hoped to be.

—**Vineet Arora, MD**, MAPP, Associate Chief Medical Officer—Clinical Learning Environment, University of Chicago Medicine

*Resilient Threads* shows why the external aims to provide better health for society cannot happen without tending to the inner imperatives. The well-being of physicians and those in the health care workforce depend on reviving joy in one's work *and* whole life. We need a holistic approach to individual courage and institutional change, and Dr. Mukta Panda shows us how it can be done.

—**Donald M. Berwick, MD**, President Emeritus and Senior Fellow, Institute for Healthcare Improvement and former Administrator, Centers for Medicare and Medicaid Services

My friend and colleague Mukta Panda has written a book straight from the heart. Mukta and I have worked together in some capacity through all the Chattanooga chapters of her life. I knew her as a young intern in the Department of Medicine who was having to repeat residency training in America, as a young faculty member, and then as even more of a colleague as she was moved up the academic ladder in the College of Medicine and became a real thought-leader on our campus. I have certainly been enriched by knowing her these many years and now by reading her book. She feels, as I do, that everything in medicine begins and ends with a patient. That's why we are here, that's why we teach, that's why we do research—it is all to provide better care to a patient. Medical students and residents reading her story will learn some of what to expect in a medical career, and for someone like me, 45-plus years into my medical and surgical career, it was an opportunity to reflect: "Oh yes, I remember feeling like that" and "Yes, this is exactly how it feels to connect to a patient." I am grateful Mukta gave us these gifts from her life experiences.

—**R. Phillip Burns, MD**, FACS, Professor and Chairman, Department of Surgery, University of Tennessee College of Medicine, Chattanooga

In a modern world of medicine where workload and the expectations of physicians are as great as they have ever been, a reminder of what makes us tick as doctors is sorely needed. This book provides that and more, from Dr. Panda's journey through her career from India to Tennessee to the encounters with individual patients that have shaped her life. As she says, patients teach us lessons that are not found in medicine textbooks, and the rich collection of these stories is inspiring and refreshing. She focuses on the relationship between physician and patient and the value that brings but is not afraid to discuss some of the bleakest situations that we can find ourselves in, from the suicide of a colleague to depression. I am a better physician for reading it.

—**Professor Andrew Goddard, MD**, FRCP (Hon), President of the Royal College of Physicians of London, consultant physician and gastroenterologist at Royal Derby Hospital

As burnout affects over half of practicing physicians and is estimated to cost the U.S. health care system $4.6 billion annually, resilience and grit become important skills for physicians in practice. Resilience is characterized by having the ability to recover from adversity and to be elastic in response to stress, whereas grit is represented by the tireless quest to reach a goal regardless of obstacles. These two ideas are different, but are closely related. Healthy physicians pursue their goals relentlessly and are able to recover quickly from adversity. In this memoir, Mukta Panda, a foreign-born MD, describes her pathway to becoming a U.S. physician (her goal) and describes ways that she has been able to put meaning into her life (resilience). The book serves as a lesson for all of us. We need to recognize our strengths and weaknesses, focus on what is important, and make sure that we have meaning in our lives. Success is measured in our ability to function as compassionate caregivers for our patients and their families.

—**Marc J. Kahn, MD**, MBA, MACP, FRCP–London, Peterman-Prosser Professor, Sr. Associate Dean, Tulane University School of Medicine; Adjunct, AB Freeman School of Business

An intimate example of how to live and work, *Resilient Threads* offers an inspiring model for others to learn from, resonate with, and be emboldened by. Dr. Mukta Panda has written a powerful and soulful human book that interweaves her experiences and action in the world of health care during her years in this sacred, imperfect, beautiful profession. It is a story that will be so very important to everyone who reads it—across every dimension of healthcare or patienthood.

—**Penelope R. Williamson**, co-author of *Leading Change in Healthcare*, Associate Professor of Medicine, The Johns Hopkins University School of Medicine

# Resilient Threads

## ALSO BY THE AUTHOR

*Rhythm of our Hearts: Philosophical Dialogue Between Father and Daughter*

Mukta Panda and Shyam Parashar

# Resilient Threads

WEAVING JOY AND MEANING
INTO WELL-BEING

## Mukta Panda, M.D.
Foreword by Timothy P. Brigham, MDiv, PhD

CREATIVE
COURAGE
PRESS

Creative Courage Press, LLC (Palisade, CO) www.CreativeCouragePress.com

**Author's note:** Stories about my work as a clinician and educator do not reflect the opinion of the University of Tennessee Health Science Center (UTHSC) College of Medicine, the UTHSC College of Medicine at Chattanooga, or its affiliate hospital. I have changed people's names and certain identifying characteristics, especially where medical histories are described. Where actual names are used, permission was granted.

This book is not intended as a substitute for the medical advice of physicians. The reader should regularly consult a physician in matters relating to one's health, particularly with symptoms that may require diagnosis or medical attention.

3M, Littmann, Master Cardiology, Classic III, and the shape of the stethoscope chestpiece are trademarks of 3M.

Brief portions of Chapter 4, Meeting Point, first appeared in "Physicians and the Power of Our 'Palms,'" Southern Medical Journal, Volume 96, Number 3, March 2003, 219. © 2003 by The Southern Medical Association.

ISBN (hardcover) 978-0-98556-654-8
ISBN (paperback) 978-0-98556-655-5
ISBN (ebook) 978-0-98556-656-2

First Edition (all formats): January 2020

Library of Congress Control Number:2019920229

Author photo by David Humber
Cover photo by Shelly L. Francis
Back cover photo by Mark Lovejoy
Cover design by Jennifer Miles Design

*Dedicated to my parents, Shyam and Shashi Parashar,*
*and my children, Natasha and Rajas, Nikhil and Anuja*

All the wisdom of the world repeats: "know yourself," "ask who you are," "enter into your inmost self," "discover your heart."

RAIMON PANIKKAR

# CONTENTS

# FOREWORD

by Timothy P. Brigham, MDiv, PhD
Chief of Staff and Chief of Education and Organizational
Development, Accreditation Council for Graduate Medical
Education (ACGME)

*In the middle of the road of my life I awoke in a wood dark
and deep, for the true way is wholly lost.*

DANTE

Becoming a physician is to embark on a lifelong journey that
starts in medical school and extends through the length of a
physician's medical career and beyond. Walking the path to
learning and practicing the art and science of medicine is
sometimes an arduous and scary task. It takes levels and years
of dedication, motivation, persistence, and relational skills that
few would be willing to commit to and far less understand. The
way is long, at times full of wonder and joy, and at times dark
and foreboding. It is a true journey of awe.

"Awe" is a word that combines twin and seemingly paradoxical concepts: a reverential sense of wonder and an intense feeling of fear and terror. That is the emotional tightrope our physicians, nurses, and other health care professional walk as they care for people in the neediest, most vulnerable, and at times, scariest moments of their lives. It can be a walk of profound awe: babies take their first breath, healings and cures that the patient views as miraculous occur, and tears are shed of gratitude and joy. It can also contain moments of awe from a different perspective: patients will take their last breath, news the physician breaks may alter the trajectory of a life, and tears of grief and despair at times rain down the cheeks of the bereaved. It takes a special person to enter this field. The roller-coaster-like trials and triumphs of the sacred healing work of a physician can be emotionally taxing during the best of times. But these do not feel like the best of times. Far from it. Far from it indeed.

Studies indicate that something has fundamentally shifted in the balance of "awe" in the lives of physicians and other members of the health care team. It is estimated that over half of physicians suffered from burnout in the United States in 2019. Depression rates for residents are higher than those of their age-matched peers. Suicide rates among physicians are the highest of any profession and significantly higher than that of the general population. There is truly an epidemic among our caregivers that is both complex and foreboding. Like Dante in the 14th century standing in a forest "dark and deep," we find ourselves in the complex ecosystem of health care lost and afraid, seeking wise and learned souls to lead us to the light.

Dr. Mukta Panda is such a person. Mukta is a healer who can confront, challenge, and change the system because she has looked within her own heart and remembered and reconnected her life with the values, connections, and passions that led her to be a physician in the first place. She knows it's possible, even necessary, to honor our complex emotions and those of the people around us in order to reclaim the humanism, professionalism, and joy in medicine. She knows because she's been there—as an educator, mother, immigrant, medical student, resident, practicing physician, faculty member, program director, department chair, and assistant dean. In all her roles she has faced numerous challenges and opportunities, and by paying attention to her heart and deeply connecting with others, she shows us a way to navigate in "unknown seas."

*Resilient Threads* takes us on a journey into the inner landscape of her life to show us a way out of "the wood dark and deep." It is a deeply personal narrative of her journey towards greater belonging, well-being, and joy. Through increasing connection, she is reigniting meaning in clinical practice, her personal life, and in system renewal. In opening up the story of her life so completely and courageously, the book resonates with wisdom and authenticity rarely seen. It demonstrates the truth and power of story—and Mukta is a master storyteller. Her story resonates in ways that goes beyond data and demonstrates that sharing vulnerability is an act of strength and may be the route to transformation in life, in work, and in the clinical working and learning environment. She shows that the effectiveness of stories is a way to learn from the past and from each other, to build trust, empathy, and compassion, and to foster well-being and joy in life and work. By sharing her stories of how she lives her life as a leader with a heart open (and sometimes broken), she lights the way forward for medical students, residents, and practicing physicians to live lives and to curate a system of medical education and health care that is patient- and family-centered and filled with well-being, joy, and belonging.

This is a must-read for learners, educators, and practicing clinicians as they journey on the path of mastery. As Desmond

Tutu illustrates in the closing quote, it will not be easy to emerge from the "wood dark and deep" without scratches, bumps, and bruises, nor without tripping and falling at times—Mukta amply illustrates that in *Resilient Threads*—but it will be worth it. There are lives at stake and treasures of joy and wonder to be found.

With this book, the path is illuminated. Dr. Panda deserves high praise and admiration for this effort. *Resilient Threads* is a gift for you as a learner, teacher or practicing physician. Read it and enjoy.

———

*Discovering more joy does not, I'm sorry to say, save us from the inevitability of hardship and heartbreak. In fact, we may cry more easily, but we will laugh more easily too. Perhaps we are just more alive. As we discover more joy, we can face suffering in a way that ennobles rather than embitters. We have hardship without becoming hard. We have heartbreak without being broken.*

DESMOND TUTU

# INTRODUCTION

*What you seek is seeking you.*

RUMI

*Who am I? Where do I belong? How do I heal as I strive to serve?*

The answers to these questions emerged over many years as I learned to reflect on the stories of my life as a physician, a mother, an immigrant. Stories can hold magic, power, and sacredness. Stories are the seeds of who we are, who we are to become, and where we belong. It is vital to recall who and what sustains us when we are struggling through difficult times. And these are difficult times.

The complex challenges in health care for me and my colleagues are taking place in a time of unprecedented change. As a physician, an educator, and a leader, I am barraged from every direction with fundamental questions about the future state of medicine. *Will all health care be remote and robotic, with human encounters only seldom? Will the cost be prohibitive? Will there be any physicians left? Will physicians be able to sustain their life force as they hold the lives of their patients?*

The well-being of a physician matters. An epidemic exists that threatens the fabric of our society, one tired and tattered physician at a time. Burnout affects not only physicians but all stakeholders, from the janitorial staff and the cafeteria workers to the nurses and students, as well as the families of those who work in health care.

Recently I was discussing with a colleague whether to do a well-being survey for our organization, the third one in three years. I was considering what questions to ask to ascertain our institution's progress toward creating a culture of well-being. Admitting he is a cynic about physician burnout, depression, stress, and suicide rates, he said, "I have my own biases. I see there is a burgeoning of literature, but the literature is in its infantile stages."

I was thinking, *Really, you say this even now?* I was remembering my dear colleague whose lifeless body I found after he died by suicide in 2016, which lit a fire within me to find the data to prove that our institution faced the same stark burnout rates. I tried a different angle, "Look, we're talking about physician engagement, which impacts patient care and quality." I could see that my point resonated with him, and I added. "It's about empowering physicians and giving them a sense of voice and agency."

He replied, "I totally agree with you. We have to communicate. I do understand moral distress, but I think it's blown out of proportion."

I responded, "It's sad that we think about these conditions superficially but we don't spend time thinking about their root causes. Just because we give a lecture on fatigue management, we think we've addressed the topic. There are things inherent to the system culture we need to look at."

Establishing a culture of well-being happens slowly, one step at a time. It often feels like five steps forward and six steps back. Culture will change at the speed of trust. What really connects people are stories. I tried to bring my argument closer to the moment. "What we're doing here right now, together, is sharing our stories. Just sharing our stories is important."

I wasn't angry at my colleague's comments. At least he was being honest with me, and we can agree to disagree without hard feelings. I respected that he felt safe to speak authentically with me. Such an open conversation would not have been possible a few years ago. It's better to know where people stand so we can move forward together.

## A Day in the Life

I am an internist, which means I tend to the large length-and-breadth field of internal medicine, from acute conditions like heart attack or stroke to long-term issues and chronic disease states like diabetes or dementia. I went to medical school in India and trained as a non-US internal medicine resident in Tennessee.

I am also a clinical educator at a teaching hospital in Chattanooga, Tennessee. Since 1998, I have provided education and patient care with a team of learners: students still in medical school and residents of medicine who are training to become independent board-certified practitioners (which for internal medicine takes three years after medical school). I supervise and teach the learners while caring for patients both in the inpatient and outpatient settings. We also admit patients from the emergency room and see those already admitted to the hospital.

I am asked to guide my teams and learners with courage, resilience, and wisdom, and to create an environment in which I myself and my learners can explore the depths of our questions around meaning and purpose:

*How do I create an environment in which I am able to retain my commitment while also openly expressing my concerns? And through it all, how do I honor my own experience and not lose sight of the core values that brought me to this vocation?*

Training in medical school and onwards mainly focuses on disease management. We seldom acknowledge that we, the caregivers, are people just like our patients. While we are training and providing care, life happens to us too. We journey through the milestones of our own maturing: financial stresses, marriage, parenting, career transitions, personal losses, health challenges, becoming caregivers of family and patients. We rarely speak about "how to live" through and in spite of our stress as human beings within our various roles.

Often it can feel like there is a disconnect, as if I'm a physician only from 8 a.m. to 8 p.m. and I should keep my parenting or family obligations to after hours. We're trained to compartmentalize. But as educators, we have to be more open about the chasm between our personal and professional lives. The learners we are guiding are living their lives, just as they are taking care of patients. It should not be taboo to bring our life issues into the workplace.

*How do medical professionals live as whole people, caring for their own health and heart?* Too often we settle for delayed gratification, saying, "When I get through medical school or residency, training eight, nine, ten or more hours of work every day, I will live my life." But this *is* our life, our work *is* living, so let us name and claim it as that and not make home and work mutually exclusive. Let us break down the barriers of our compartments and live a connected and joined life.

Recognizing the disservice of reinforcing the professional-personal disconnect, I decided to initiate a "How to Live" curriculum at my institution. Such a program of studies was certainly not included in any of the educational institutions I have attended.

Instead, "How to Live" names, claims, and nurtures the inner life of physicians by making time to reflect on our practice of medicine as real people living real lives. Reflection was ingrained in my culture in India, although I often called it meditation. In Hindi, we called it *dhyaan,* which means to "be in thought." I saw the power in witnessing my grandfather meditating every morning. I felt the power in my own journal writing every night to think about my day, what happened, and what I could learn from it. These days I describe my practice as being intentional.

It is not only that we need to take care of ourselves. We also need to reclaim our purpose, our reason for choosing the call of medicine, and connect our purpose to that passion, which is to care for our patients.

## We Can't Stereotype Human Life

Textbooks of medicine teach and emphasize the physical aspects of what a disease does to the patient. We are taught from our first days to stereotype symptoms. Left-sided exertional chest pain radiating to the left arm or jaw strongly indicates the possibility of heart ischemia or heart attack. The sudden inability to talk, with weakness on one side of the body, indicates the possibility of a stroke, and so on. Stereotyping can lead to bias and premature conclusions.

Medicine is more than care of a patient's disease; we are also caring for the person in which disease, illness, or injury has occurred. Here is an example I often share with my students that illustrates the difference.

In today's health care system, hospitals track quality metrics like length of stay and readmission rate of patients. Physicians work in shifts of seven days on, seven off, and so a patient may see two or three physicians during their hospital stay. Their care often feels disjointed, in need of coordination for continuity. Imagine a patient who comes in with hypertension and is treated for that, then released. Repeated admissions for that person's hypertension counts against the physician and the hospital. Let us look beyond metrics. How can we get to the story of why a patient is readmitted again and again?

Around 2010, a woman in her fifties kept coming back to the hospital with the same complaints almost every month for a year. Each time she had very high blood sugars due to uncontrolled diabetes from not taking insulin. The night team admitted her and handed her off to our team the next morning, saying "This patient is here again. She just needs her insulin and we can discharge her." I went to see the patient, but she was curled up fast asleep, with her food tray untouched next to the bed. It was a very busy day, so I left to go visit other patients and tried again later. Every time I went back during my shift, she was still asleep. On the second day, I went by again and again, but she was still asleep. It seemed very strange because her parameters and vital signs looked fine, so I knew she was okay. She just looked tired.

By early evening, forty-eight hours into her stay, I decided to intervene. It was time to uncover her story. I woke her up. "Hello. I'm Dr. Panda. Are you feeling better? Are you still feeling very tired?" She nodded, and I continued. "I really would like to know what brought you to the hospital. Would you mind sitting up so we can have a conversation?" The woman reluctantly sat up in bed.

I pulled up the blinds. "There's still a little daylight. It's a beautiful scene outside. Are you hungry?" I could stop the glucose drip if she would start eating. "Once we see you're awake and can stop your IV fluids, we can discharge you back home from the hospital."

"I'm not hungry," she said.

"Well, tell me how long have you had diabetes. How can I help you?" That's how we began our conversation. I sat and listened.

I learned that she worked at a Waffle House. She had developed a nonhealing ulcer on her foot, for which a podiatrist had prescribed antibiotics, but it didn't heal. Her primary care physician told her that she needed to be off her foot or she would lose it. She had taken a few days off of work, but then lost her job. That led to her moving in with her son and daughter-in-law, becoming an unpaid babysitter for her three grandchildren. Because she still had to pay rent, she had no money to buy her insulin. Now I could see the bigger picture. She was coming to the hospital for respite.

"Look, why don't you get something to eat. Would you like to have some visitors?" She shook her head.

"We have a team, including chaplains and case managers, who are available to talk with people about coping. Would you like that?" She nodded. "I'll have them come first thing in the morning and I will send my medical student, too." I didn't want to bombard her with all my questions at the same time.

At rounds the next morning, I told my team, "I think there's more to her story. She may need some support from social services. She was working at Waffle House until a few weeks ago. It looks like she cannot afford her medicine. Try to get some more information about that, then we can talk more about it. And be gentle with her." They always laugh when I remind them to be gentle. The team went in and took more history. She was more awake. I spoke to the nurse, "Keep the window blinds open. See if she'd like to shower, and kindly make sure she eats."

Later that day I visited her again with the chaplain and a student. I said, "Thank you so much for the earlier conversations. Now we have a better understanding of how we can help you." I shared the opportunities available and asked, "What do you suggest?"

"I really want to go back to work. I enjoy my work. I don't know if I want to go back to *that* place, but I do want to work."

I reassured her, "We can give you a certificate to prove to your employer that you need medical rest and medical leave."

"Doctor, I don't know if it will help or not."

I was reminded how many people lack a safety net. They have only so much flexibility in their life and that's it. I requested more assistance from the chaplains, case manager, and legal aid. With their help, she was able to get her job back.

I saw her again about three months later at the outpatient clinic. She had a new job, a place of her own to live, new clothes, and was even wearing pink nail polish. She said to me, "You don't recognize me, do you, doctor!" I replied with a big smile, "No, I don't!"

This story shows what I mean when I say we must treat patients, not the disease. It was nearly a year before she was readmitted to the hospital. She came instead to the clinic for routine treatment and help. Yes, we extended that specific hospital stay by a few extra days to find out more about her life, but over time we helped the whole person that she is *and* saved the system thousands of dollars by getting to the root of her problem. We had initially stereotyped her as a noncompliant "frequent flyer" patient, but that was not it. We just had to ask and listen.

Experiences like this encourage my students to strive mindfully to build relationships by viewing our patients as human beings, or even as spiritual beings who happen to be in a human body. The initial human connection we establish will help us care for each patient in a much more mutually meaningful and fulfilling way. It is through those relationships that our patients can teach us to cope and to thrive despite adversities and vulnerabilities.

This case happened about nine months into a grant project for integrating clinically trained chaplains into our internal medicine training program. As part of the program evaluation, I shared her story with the leadership. The value of the chaplain's empathy and compassion and the resulting economic savings was clearly evident. We were able to continue the funding that would allow the chaplains to remain onboard as faculty.[1]

This patient story—and many more in Parts Two and Three —also illustrates the difference between routine (attending to disease in a patient) and ritual (intending to discover the story of a person). Disease in a living person doesn't behave as it does in a textbook, or even the same way in each unique individual. So many factors influence a disease and a patient's outcome. For the best results, we need to combine both the data of evidence-based medicine with the stories of empathy-based medicine.

## May Ritual Become Our Routine

I believe in following the ritual of medicine. As soon as you introduce yourself to a patient, and stretch out your hand in your white coat, that patient is completely naked—physically, emotionally, spiritually. We see humanity at its most vulnerable times. Ritual is created in how we take the history and perform the first physical exam. We are trained to ask, "What brings you to the hospital?" A template is drilled into the minds of first-year students. It goes into the records of the patient; as you take his or her story (history), you must get to know that person and establish their trust. The template routine feels like such a checklist! I tell my students, don't think of this as a template but as a ritual.

A ritual has a personal intentionality and mindfulness. I brush my teeth every day as a routine, but when I pray in the morning it's a ritual. Getting dressed every day is routine, but when I'm attending a special occasion I have a different ritual. Eating alone at my computer is a routine (not that it's the right thing to do!), but eating with my family is a ritual.

A kind bedside manner results from ritual, not a routine. Instead of asking, "What's bothering you today?" I like to start by saying, "I'm Dr. Panda, I look forward to getting to know you," or "How can I help you?" I have even asked anxious-appearing adolescent patients, "What's your favorite ice cream?" If I'm speaking to a grandparent, I ask about grandkids. I try not to stare at the computer or a sheet. I make and hold eye-to-eye contact. I try to be mindful of my own visceral body reactions, like increased heart rate or a tightness in my jaw or shoulders. When someone comes in disheveled, I try not to stereotype them versus someone who walks in wearing a suit and tie. I know I have unconscious biases, as we all do. If someone is fighting for their life, I try to discern and be mindful of how are they coping. How can I relate and find some level of connection with what they are going through or have been through?

Routine steps happen without intentionality, more out of habit than choice. Routine feels superficial, but ritual connects our passion with purpose, our soul to our role. When we practice medicine in a ritualistic fashion, we connect *who* we are with *what* we do and *how* we do it. Ritual can be as simple as taking time to be silent, but if you just say "I'm going to take a lie down" and your head is still whirling, you're not really resting. That's still multitasking in a hundred directions. Instead, you put your whole self into resting. That's hard for me, even today. It takes practice.

Ritual, relationships, and reflection are key threads in how I learned to thrive. *What if we made more effort to learn from each other about the entirety of who we are and who we teach, who we connect with day to day? What if reflecting on our lives—and sharing those insights—were part of our teaching and role modeling?* Perhaps the next generation of physicians will be more resilient because they will not wait decades into their career (like I did) to gain strength through self-awareness and story-sharing.

Whenever I orient a new team, I name the importance of questions, "I ask a lot of questions—and I answer most of them. Questions are how I think and how I reason." I give them an invitation up front, "I want you to always ask a lot of questions. One of the most important words for you in medicine is *why*. If you don't understand the *why*, you will not know how to treat the patient."

It's harder to answer questions related to culture change or personal growth. Rhetorical questions can cause frustration in those who want answers and in those who are expected to have all the answers. But some questions inspire ongoing reflection. I am reminded of the poet Rainer Maria Rilke who advised his young protégé: [2]

> I want to beg you, as much as I can, dear sir, to be patient toward all that is unsolved in your heart and to try to love the questions themselves like locked rooms and like books that are written in a very foreign tongue. Do not now seek the answers, which cannot be given you because you would not be able to live them. And the point is, to live everything. Live the questions now. Perhaps you will then gradually, without noticing it, live along some distant day into the answer.

It's uncomfortable to have unanswered questions. It's important to surrender and say to yourself, "I don't need to have *all* the answers as long as I can live into the questions and hold the tension for what it is, to be comfortable with not knowing." For me, there is so much peace in that. But that's a lesson that came with hindsight.

## May My Stories Serve

It was hard for me to write this book. There was a fear of risking my livelihood, risking the persona that people may have of me. But trust is more authentic than fear. I trust that the stories shared here might give voice to two main themes of my ongoing life journey: *returning human touch to health care* and *respecting the whole person*, whether patient, medical student, resident, friend, family member, colleague, or physician. My stories emphasize spirituality and the sacredness crucial to human relationships.

I hope in particular to address and give voice to two groups that face overwhelming and unrelieved stress: *exhausted health care professionals* burdened with unprecedented responsibilities separate from patient care, and *women* caught in fatiguing mazes of complexity as they endeavor to integrate and balance life demands across roles, functions, and cultures in our fragmented world. There remains a real and formidable glass ceiling for women in both medicine and academia.

I have often pondered the poem "The Way It Is" by William Stafford.[3] He talks about the thread you follow, which doesn't change even as it goes among things that change. I visualize my stories as a tapestry woven from their many threads added, cut, joined, entangled, and intersected over the years. These threads are soft, coarse, harsh, silken, fragile, and strong. They all have a place and a purpose. Some of these threads were given to me by my family, friends, my culture, religion, tradition, professions, and society. Many threads I have collected intentionally, many more unconsciously, and some have even been collected unwillingly. The undersurface is uneven, knotted, and ugly in parts.

Through all of life, we each have at least one abiding thread. For me it is the braided hope and faith that life has beauty, and that if you believe in a higher power—I call it God

—we will not only survive but thrive. I have attempted to thrive in spite of the messy undersurface. Some parts of life must be dealt with under the surface in order to allow the beautiful picture to rise to the top.

Today there are parts of my life I prefer not to speak about in detail, even though I accept that they are both the beautiful and painful parts. Terry Tempest Williams, in her book *When Women Were Birds*,[4] reflected that we must discern when to speak our truth publicly or keep the words of our heart private. She writes, "There is comfort in keeping what is sacred inside us not as a secret, but as a prayer."

My spoken and unspoken stories woven together create the beautiful tapestry landscape story of me, of who I am and where I belong. I am proud of me, with humility and gratitude to all who have been so vital in contributing to my story. These stories can inspire, sustain, call, and sometimes judge and condemn me. They are foundational to the micro and macro culture of my community of belonging.

I've learned the importance of having a community of kindred spirits to help us see the meaning of our experiences. Sharing our stories with others is a way of reflecting on our lives, building empathy, and trust. We can make sense of our purpose and learnings. I would never have seen all these connections if I were not intentional about invoking (and evoking) memories through the conversations while writing this book. Sharing our stories in community is so important!

I tell my stories through my own lens, memories and feelings. Stories about my work as a clinician and educator do not reflect the opinion of the University of Tennessee Health Science Center (UTHSC) College of Medicine, the UTHSC College of Medicine at Chattanooga, or its affiliate hospital. I have changed people's names and certain identifying characteristics, especially where medical histories are described. Where actual names are used, permission was granted.

I have learned that when dealing with the heart and emotions, there is no right or wrong. I hope you will read and absorb my stories with curiosity and kindness, and perhaps reflect on your own stories. I ask for forgiveness and understanding if anyone feels hurt or offended. This book is a way to offer gratitude for my life journey, for the people who walk with me, and for those I have encountered along the way.

More than a memoir or chronology of my career, my stories reveal the arc of rediscovering who I am, while recommitting myself daily to the well-being of patients and the students, residents, and colleagues I work with. I found the courage to share my story in hope that it resonates because it is a story of community well-being.

*The pattern should be clear. When serenity comes up out of anxiety, joy out of depression, hope out of hopelessness; when good is returned for evil, forgiveness replaces retaliation and courage triumphs over fear; then we recognize the movement of something beyond the personality and mental health. Such profound manifestations of the human spirit are the faces of the fourth dimension, which I have called the Holy.*

JAMES E. LODER

# PART 1

# WHO AM I?

*At first sight, joy seems to be connected with being different. When you receive a compliment or win an award, you experience the joy of not being the same as others. You are faster, smarter, more beautiful, and it is that difference that brings you joy. But such joy is very temporary. True joy is hidden where we are the same as other people: fragile and mortal. It is the joy of belonging to the human race. It is the joy of being with others as a friend, a companion, a fellow traveler.*

HENRI J. M. NOUWEN

# 1 WHERE ARE YOU FROM?

*If you don't know the trees you may be lost in the forest, but
if you don't know the stories you may be lost in life.*

SIBERIAN ELDER

"WHERE ARE YOU FROM?" A very simple question, but like many things, the simple questions have complicated answers. I have been asked this question numerous times over my five decades of life. Initially I often responded, "India, of course!"

However, over the past decade and a half, I have wondered what that question really means. Is it my country of origin? That would be India. Or is it where I spent most of my first five years of growing up? Well then, that would have to be London.

What about where I did my schooling and my graduate school, medical school, and transitional year residency training? That would be India again.

Or perhaps where my children were born? Saudi Arabia. Where have I spent the most years of my life, over a quarter of a century, completed my third residency in internal medicine, and continue my work as a physician educator? That's in Tennessee.

Where do I come from? It's not the same as asking *Where do I belong*? I have come to realize that it is not so much about a geographic location, but about what is inside me. Where I belong is where I feel I can become myself, where I can be who I am. Belonging is not where I am going, or where I have come from, but where I stand. The stories of my experiences frame the answer to that question. It is about what I carry within me.

I am a physician who comes from two physicians. Both my mother and father were in medical school in India when their families arranged for them to become engaged. They met for the first time on their wedding day. After a week of wedding receptions, my mother returned to her parent's home in Bhopal to finish two years of medical school, eventually graduating at the top of her class. My father continued at Gwalior Medical College (about seven hours away from my mother by train) to finish his master's degree in surgery. I was born two years later in New Delhi. It was a prolonged labor, and my father waited the whole night on a stone bench in the hospital park. For the first fifteen months of my life, my grandparents helped care for me while my parents started their careers in Delhi. My father joined the cardiothoracic department of the All India Institute of Medical Sciences, and my mother joined the pediatrics department at Irwin Hospital.

In August 1964 my parents flew to London to continue their medical specialization training, leaving me with my grandparents. I was reunited with my parents a year later, when my grandfather took me and my aunt (six years older) to England. Of course, I have no vivid memory of these years, only vague impressions of my brother being born and my fifth birthday party. We returned to India, and it wasn't long before my father became an assistant professor of surgery and my mother became an assistant professor of medicine, the faculty positions of their dreams. They worked at Goa Medical College and government hospital, the only teaching hospital offering free health care for the people of Goa.

You could say that I come from Panjim, the capital city of Goa. It feels like an old medieval European city because it was a Portuguese colony until the 1960s. On the southwestern coast, Goa also feels like the Hawaii of India, with beautiful beaches, a fishing community, and very friendly people. There are beggars and poverty, too, but it feels nothing like Bombay or Delhi. Goa's culture was a mixture of South American Brazilian cultures, a lot of partying and the carnival, and at the same time, very traditional festivals of India and the Roman Catholics. I went to a Catholic school run by nuns, going to midnight mass and volunteering at their orphanage. Growing up in Goa was heavenly.

Because my parents were on the faculty at the medical college and not in private practice, we were a middle-class family. We lived in a three-bedroom apartment, one of six such units surrounding a common courtyard. We always knew our neighbors, and borrowing a potato or a cup of sugar was commonplace. My grandmother, two brothers, and live-in house helpers completed our household. We had several different house helpers over the years. They were young girls who stayed with us until they were of age to be married. They lived in a little room behind the kitchen and we all cooked together. It was small! While this arrangement was normal in Indian culture, house helpers were like family members in our home, which was decidedly not typical. Our Hindi dialect has two forms of address when speaking to people, in lieu of the all-purpose *you* in English. "Aap" is for someone held in respect or who occupies a position or station higher than yourself. "Tum" is for a person considered below you in status or class. My parents spoke with house helpers using the respectful "Aap" and insisted we children did too.

Typically, about 5:30 p.m. after tea, grandmothers and children would collect in the courtyard where there were swings, a garden, and a badminton court. People would play and gather together. Helpers from all the flats would get together and talk. In India the caste system is ingrained and going against any grain takes considerable courage. Our way of relating to and with the house helpers in our home did not go unnoticed by other families in the community. My parents were on occasion chastised for "spoiling" our house helpers.

One day our helper named Vijaya was wearing a sari my mother had given her, and another helper noticed with jealousy that it was flashier than what others had.

"Yes, Memsaab gave it to me," Vijaya said.

"Yeah, my memsaab says your memsaab tries to show off and it's not right."

"No, no, she's very nice and kind."

Later that evening Vijaya told my mom. "I don't think I should I wear this, people are talking." My mother replied, "We shouldn't worry about what people think."

What gave my father and mother the courage to stand in another person's place and to speak for a more just way of being? For one thing, my parents were (and are) voracious readers. They also possessed a level of unusual foresight and maturity, and they traveled abroad. Throughout my childhood I was accepted as I was and encouraged to be with others of different backgrounds and religious cultures. Many people of varying backgrounds were constantly visiting our home. This was enriching for our minds and souls.

Once we had a helper of the Islamic faith who, instead of being served on a separate plate as was the prevalent custom, ate from the same set of dishes. I recall in particular both of my grandmothers being open and accepting of Muslim traditions. This, too, made a significant impression on me. Our house helpers ate what we ate, not the leftovers which were served in some other households. If there was a treat, such as Coca Cola or chocolates, we all shared equally. Each person's birthday was acknowledged with a special celebration.

Making the choice to do the right thing is commendable. Choosing to do the right thing for the right reasons makes all the difference in the world. My parents showed me how to make the right choices through the way they quietly and purposefully lived. In that daily living I learned the importance of standing for something larger than myself.

I remember one afternoon when I was eleven years old, my mother and I, as well as our young house helper, Habiba, dressed up to go to the movies. I had put on two necklaces that my mother had bought for me. I can still picture the one that had brown and maroon beads with gold-colored rings in the center. My mother said, "Why don't you wear one and give the other to Habiba. It will look so pretty with her dress." I very much wanted to keep both necklaces. Habiba was my age and beautiful. I was a little jealous. She was slim, whereas I always suffered from a weight problem as a child, my chubby puppy fat. However, I would not dream of being disagreeable and most reluctantly gave the second necklace to our house helper. Thus it was, in such subtle and gentle ways, my parents role-modeled and molded me to value and recognize everyone. It was wonderful the way my parents taught respect of all humanity.

## Following in Their Footsteps

My father's grandfather had been a *Vaidya*, an Indian tradi-tional medicine practitioner during the same years when he exchanged his usual turban and began wearing Gandhi's cap. He never charged his patients in monetary terms, not even during years of political struggle that led to financial hard-ships. My great-grandfather's patients paid with gifts of vegetables and other food. Their gifts were welcome and of great help.

During my childhood I noted how people greeted my parents as Doctor Sahib, meaning Doctor Sir, which imparted the respect they had garnered. As a young child, I didn't understand the details of their conversations but I felt the responsibility in their voices when they spoke about their work with their friends who were also physicians. They were often asked to consult about the health of their friends, neighbors, or children. I watched how my parents gave of themselves and their resources generously; everybody was so grateful to them.

My parents practiced medicine in the academic setting and strived to maintain their values of hard work, ethics, and honesty. My preteen years coincided with a time when the doctor profession was undergoing change. Physicians were still recognized to be part of that noble profession, but private practice and medicine as a business endeavor was becoming more popular in our home town. The elaborate trips, cars, and scooters given to the parents of some of my school friends were very different compared to the humble gifts of freshly home-baked bread and cakes, home-grown vegetables, and knitted scarves that my parents sometimes received. These friends no longer walked or took the bus with me, but rode in chauffeur-driven cars and went to private schools. Unsure of the reason for this discrepancy, I asked my parents one day in an almost undermining condescending way, "You must not be doing your job well and perhaps are not very good physicians. How come you don't get the same gifts as my friends' parents who are also physicians?"

My mother held my hand and said, "But of course, I do get the best gifts. When my patients look at me and say, 'God bless you' or 'Thank you' or when students that I taught years ago recognize me in spite of my gray hair now, that's the best gift."

That conversation has remained etched in me, and I remind

myself often of the core purpose of my vocation. My purpose comes not from the materialistic gifts I receive but from the relationships developed with other human beings.

I believe, as my father shared on many occasions, we come to this earth with blessings bestowed upon us by our ancestors and our previous lives (*sanchit* karma), we gather blessings through deeds we perform with integrity in our vocation (*arjit* karma), and we receive blessings from other people (*arpit* karma). These blessings are the true wealth we have, not the materialistic things. We deposit these blessings in our spiritual bank account, and we should amass enough in this bank so our children and their children will continue to be blessed.

As I grew up, I saw my parents receive and bestow such blessings. Their students came to our home, having exciting and intelligent conversations, being taught with patience. I remember my father orienting his new fellowship trainees at the beginning of their postgraduate training. He proceeded to discuss and role model the technical aspects of working in the operating room, and then he shared in a serious but compassionate voice, "...and after the patient is prepped and we are ready to begin, with the scalpel in my hand, I say a silent prayer before I start." This is a literal example of an instrument in God's hands! Because my parents seemed so fulfilled and respected and always helping others, becoming a physician like them was always in the back of my mind.

During high school I was drawn to the science of biology and human psychology, more so than to physics and chemistry. In India you go to high school through the tenth grade, then enter two years of what we called college. The educational path in India was quite restrictive in the late 1970s when I was applying for college. We could choose from only three main tracks: science, art, or commerce. For medicine or engineering, the two most highly regarded professions, we went the science route. I felt medicine was the most suitable profession for me.

Applicants had to be among the top 35 by merit to be considered. It took a lot of hard work, but I got in.

There was one final hurdle. Mummy sat me down for a frank conversation about the challenges of being a female and being a physician, especially in India. Even though it's a maternalistic society, women are responsible for the rearing of children and household management, while men have the role of the breadwinner.

"If you really want to do it, do it. It's a very gratifying job. We'll support you in whatever you want to do. But there are other options if you want."

It wasn't a long, drawn-out conversation. I simply replied, "This is the only thing I want to do."

I was sixteen and it was the monsoon season in June when I began attending Goa Medical College. I continued living at home, which was quite the norm in India. People rarely left home to attend college. I enjoyed every aspect of it—good friends and lots of competition. Our final year was very, very tough. The final year also determined what specialty you would go into. I was quite stressed out. I remember convincing my mom to let me move into campus housing. "You know, everybody who stays in the hostel, they seem to have all this time to study. I've got too many distractions at home. I'm going to go live there."

My mom said, "Look, it's going to be tough. You know, here you have somebody who cooks your food and does your laundry and makes your bed. You just have to study and do nothing else. But if you do want to go, go."

I packed up my suitcase and left. I came back two days later. She never said a word. After that I advised everybody, "Don't ever go, just stay at home. It's paradise."

## Taking the Next Expected Step

During college, I never made up my mind as to what specialty I wanted to pursue. I just wanted to become a physician. I thought medical education—being an educator of medical professionals—is what I should do because that's what I saw my parents do. After I finished medical school and took my qualifying exam, I got married, which was simply the next logical step in the life of a girl growing up in India.

My future depended on where married life would take me. The two of us never had a specific talk about our life together. It was simply understood that where he went, I would follow. The wedding was in December 1984. By September the next year I was pregnant.

—

*The farthest horizons of our hopes and fears are cobbled by our poems, carved from the rock experiences of our daily lives.*

AUDRE LORDE

## 2  THE GIFT OF GENERATIONS

*The great secret of true success, of true happiness, is this: the man or woman who asks for no return, the perfectly unselfish person, is the most successful.*

SWAMI VIVEKANANDA

BEFORE PROCEEDING with stories of becoming a mother and a physician myself, I feel I must loop the thread of my life back to the stories of my parents' parents. Their lives influenced who I became. Their values influence the tapestry of life I aspire to weave for my own children. My three grandparents were very nurturing, encircling me with grace and simplicity. How we show up in the world depends a lot on where we came from, where we can be comfortable, how we are welcomed, and where we can be authentic and belong.

The grandparent-grandchild relationship is special and can play an important role in the development of our personality and behavior. I was blessed with grandparents who are still my life-long role models of discipline, perseverance in hard times, courage, and faith. The education my grandparents gave me was really a How to Live curriculum.

## A Woman of Few Words

*Our fingerprints don't fade from the lives we touch.*

JUDY BLUME

Naniji, my maternal grandmother, was widowed at a young age when my grandfather died of a massive heart attack while walking to his office one autumn morning. I was a baby and had only spent a day with him. In an instant, Naniji went from being a wife, thus an honored person in the existing social structure, to someone with no individual identity. She now found herself with a daughter (my mother) and two sons to raise alone. From the day of my grandfather's death, she removed the *bindi* from her forehead which had identified her as a married woman, and she never wore fancy jewelry again. For the rest of her long life, her sari was white, the color for mourning. For Naniji, these were acts of devotion, submission, and true humility. She not only acknowledged Indian customs and traditions, but also deeply believed them to be right.

My earliest memory of Naniji was from around the age of five. She wore her life with grace and strength, and with a dignity that continues to inspire me to this day. That rock-solid faith shaped her hours, days, months, and years in ways that were not always tangible or reasonable to me as a child. Her unfailing habit of rising at 4 a.m. to shower in cold water, for example, or her total silence until she had prayed for an hour and a half each morning, and again for an hour in the evening by lamp light, were curious to my young, practical mind. Once I challenged her as being old-fashioned by asking, "Naniji, why are you praying?" This woman of few words responded from her heart, "Why, I pray for you! For your brothers, and for your parents—for all the family, their health and happiness always."

"What about you? Do you not pray for yourself? What is your prayer for you?" I responded.

"I just ask God to take me while I am walking and independent," was her immediate unhindered reply. Her words touched me profoundly, and I still hold them in my heart as I pray daily for my own family.

My grandmother departed from one important custom, however, which speaks of her extraordinary inner strength. She maintained her home in Bhopal, a two-day train journey from us in Goa. Nanaji kept house frugally and independently on a small pension from my grandfather's years with the railroad company and with some help from her two sons. She made it very clear that her greatest desire was to not become a burden on anyone. Outwardly she followed tradition by moving through the days quietly and staying close to her home, seldom going to community events or celebrations. Most social gatherings required married status, and since she had chosen independence over living with her parents or her in-laws, there were few events where she *fit in* and even fewer where she could *belong*. Tradition dictated that once a widow, always a widow; following that, the question of remarrying simply did not arise. My grandmother was acting on her values, rather than the societal norm, therefore remaining true to herself with her integrity intact.

Uneducated in the formal sense, my soft-spoken Naniji was both a master at the art of living in peace with courage and conviction, as well as the matriarch who kept our family together. Naniji would come from Bhopal to Goa to live with us for a few weeks during the times my mother needed her help to care for me and my two younger brothers. When I would open my schoolbooks at home, she would study English alongside me or work on a crochet or knitting project. The fragrant, complex dishes she cooked for us were always served with a large portion of love.

Naniji's guidance was strict, particularly when we would go out in public. She paid attention to our attire, and we felt prompted to follow her firm direction, not out of mute obedience, but as a response to her love. Our grandmother nudged us to think and act from a sense of knowing the correct thing to do. Knowing very well from experience what opposition to cultural norms was like, she was nonetheless undeterred from being a role model to me. Everything she said and did was thoughtful and with purpose; her economy of words unfailingly spoke volumes.

One day, I gained a little insight to my grandmother's sense of humor when I became gripped with a severe case of hiccups. We were sitting together on the divan in our apartment. She was stitching away on a piece of fabric, head down, absorbed with her task. In the middle of my hiccup attack, she said, "I'm really disappointed. If you are upset with me you should talk with *me* instead of going behind my back and talking with your aunt." Shocked, I burst out, "I never said anything! What are you talking about? That is not true!" Then with a mischievous smile playing in her eyes, she quipped, "The hiccups are gone, aren't they?" Indeed they were, and we had a good laugh over her strategy. Today I still remember this remedy and use it with delight on my friends and family.

Naniji was not educated in academic studies, but oh, was she schooled in the ways of wisdom. Without actually thinking about it, I gradually absorbed lessons by watching and listening while she carried out the rhythmic tasks of the day. As Naniji cuddled my baby brother, we would have little one-on-one talks. One particular talk continues to prove invaluable. I remember being upset about something a friend had told another friend about me. I was hurt and told Naniji about the episode. She in her wise demeanor listened and then calmly shared, "Mukta, God has given us all a tongue. It will wag irrespective if you do good or do bad. When to let it wag is in our control and the choice we have to make. Use it to praise and lift up others. If you cannot say anything good about others, it is better to keep quiet."

Many times her words have been poignant reminders for me! Such wisdom gained from those times with my grandmother has stayed with me throughout my life. She taught me the invaluable lesson that a person does not need letters or a title in front of her name to impart knowledge and understanding or to shape a child's moral and ethical fiber.

At the end of Naniji's visits to us in Goa, my uncle would come to pick her up. We always made a follow-up plan as to when we'd see her again. We repeated the same scene. The night before she left, I would cry, "Why do you have to go back? Why can't you stay with us?" and she would always reply, "I will come back and you will come visit me."

A tradition in India before anyone leaves your home is to give them enough food to cover their journey. We'd pack *puris* (a type of Indian bread) and vegetables that would not spoil over a two-day train ride. We would do *Tika,* which means to put a small mark of red powder called *sindoor* on the traveler's forehead and give them an offering of something sweet to eat. At the doorstep, the younger generation would also touch the feet of the older generation to receive their blessings. When an older person bids goodbye to a younger person, they often give an offering of cash. Naniji would hand each of us a roll of rupees, in different amounts but always ending in 1 (such as 51, 101, 201, 251, and so on), with that one extra rupee for blessings and good luck. While it was nice to receive that money, we handed the cash to our parents. Naniji would give my parents more cash than us children.

This was Naniji's way of "paying back" her daughter, as

parents were not expected to be burdens to their married daughters who now belonged to another family. Widows were usually cared for in their son's household. With her personal presence she showered us with so much emotionally and intellectually, as well as physically with special treats that she cooked.

During summer vacations from the academic year, I would travel to visit Naniji in her own surroundings in Bhopal. Her home had lots of open space for us to explore. The kitchen was the clean and sacred space. The stove was lit only after my grandmother finished her morning shower. I remember a pantry in the back of her kitchen where my grandmother stored all the delicious mango pickles she made for the year, which were some of my favorite. She made the raw mangoes and lemon ooze with amazing spices and aroma while maintaining their unique taste—pure delicious goodness. No one has been able to duplicate the flavor of her mouthwatering pickles.

Having enjoyed robust health well into her eighties, there came a time when she suffered from both osteoporosis and osteoarthritis. After a hard fall which broke her hip, she was bedridden for about a year. My aunts, uncles, and cousins willingly and lovingly took care of her needs, including bathing and toileting. During her life my grandmother requested only two things—hot, hot tea and crisp toast in the morning and evening. Eventually, she could not accept the dependency her condition required and stopped eating or drinking in order to spare others the burden of cleaning up. Dependency had been her worst fear and her prayer was to be spared from it.

I arranged flights from the US specifically to be with her, only to be questioned upon my arrival about why I was there. She would say, "You should be spending time with your family. I'm okay and have lots of people looking after me." That was my Naniji, never thinking of herself, only others. The last time she said this, I laughed with her through my tears, knowing the end of her life was coming. Because Naniji lived a fine balance between courage and flexibility, she indirectly passed this practice to her grandchildren.

After Grandmother left this world, my family found a paper on which she had written her will. Not one of us was forgotten. The names on the paper included even her grandchildren's spouses. Every family member received an item that carried her love forward. Naniji gave me her set of silver deity, which were in her puja. She knew I followed a ritual of puja, or prayer, in my own life. I still have them in the center of my prayer room, inside the same round steel box she gave me. To the last, she remained true to her character, giving everything of herself to others.

## A Peaceful Presence

> *The true mysteries of life accomplish themselves so softly,
> with so easy and assured a grace, so frank an acceptance
> of our breeding, striving, dying, unresting world, that the
> unimaginative man is hardly startled by their daily and
> radiant revelation of infinite wisdom and love.*

EVELYN UNDERHILL

You would be hard-pressed to find a person more genuine and content with life than my paternal grandmother. Her courage was the type based upon quiet acceptance, grace, and submission to those life events over which she had no control.

Dadiji came to live with us for months at a time when I was growing up in Goa, thus my experiences with her were plentiful. Several of my grandmother's remarkable qualities stand out in memory, such as her quiet nature, her thoughtful words when speaking of others, and her pure love for family. To my knowledge, she never asked for anything or complained about her situation. Dressing simply and dwelling happily at home, it seemed as if it never crossed her mind to be disgruntled about details.

Dadiji did not even require a chair, but sat instead on the floor, as was the custom in India. She preferred eating meals while sitting on the floor as well, and rarely consented to go out to restaurants. One year on my father's birthday, after much discussion and persuasion from my brother and myself, we decided to celebrate at a restaurant. This was truly against tradition and norms in our family—dinner was typically held at home with all of us, nearby or visiting relatives, and occasionally a close family friend. Sharing this decision of a family treat, I exclaimed to Dadiji, "Let's go out to eat at the hotel! Wear a new sari! Dress up!" Afterward, I asked if she had not enjoyed the outing. Thoughtfully she replied, "Well...it wasn't like we celebrate at home, with our sweetmeats." This was the nearest thing she ever said to me that resembled a negative comment! Dadiji thoroughly relished a good meal complete with plenty of rich variety and sweet treats, but, for her, home was the place for body and soul no matter what the occasion.

Stories of her childhood filled my grandmother's heart with happiness, and she was fond of relating them to me while chewing on her one luxury, tobacco. Her lap was soft and cuddly, and with her beautiful smile Dadiji would speak lovingly of the ways her grandparents and her parents, especially her father, doted on her. According to her firsthand account, she was a pampered child who never once suffered in all her years. She spoke about her grandfather sneaking sweet treats for her when no one was looking. As she spoke, I imagined a younger Dadiji, smiling, without a care in the world, skipping along in the fields with her friends, *Sakhis* as she called them. Without bragging, which was not in her nature, she simply stated the facts as she remembered them. Never did I hear her utter a criticism or make an unkind remark about another person.

I remember the summer holiday when I was fourteen. I was trying to keep track of my two-year-old brother who was dashing gleefully around the apartment as lunch was being prepared. Dadiji, who sat in her customary place on the floor, wanted no food, only water. She had not felt well for a day or so. Returning to her with the glass of water, I caught a glimpse of my little brother as he bolted outside, so I left my grandmother and ran out after him. When I came back just a few minutes later, my Dadiji was slumped over, the water spilling beside her.

This was my first encounter with death. With feelings of pure panic and fear, I screamed for my parents. I remember the pain on their faces. I saw my father cry for the first time. I remember crowds of people in our small three-bedroom apartment. By the time my grandfather, aunts, and uncles arrived a few days later, Dadiji's body had already been cremated according to tradition. Relatives from America came, and on the thirteenth day after her death, also in keeping with the convention, we held her ceremony. Each person chose something to remember my grandmother by, and then quite suddenly they were gone. I kept her holy book, the *Ramayana*, from which she used to read daily. I continue to read from it today.

People have said that I carry qualities from both of my grandmothers, namely acceptance from Dadiji and generosity from Naniji. I have generally accepted life as it is with unconditional faith. My grandmothers were content in the same way. I strive to be happy, in peace, and free of fear. This unconditional acceptance and lack of curiosity in my personal life strikes me as paradoxical when compared to my professional life in which no stone is left unturned, no clue left unexamined in the quest for solutions to health care issues. Perhaps I need to consider this conundrum further, but then again, perhaps not. For now, I am content to live with the question.

## Sacred Threads

> *Talk that matters comes from lives that matter. Seldom does meaningful talk issue from a chaotic life. The chaos demands too much attention, interrupts almost every conversation, and trivializes talk that otherwise might matter. There are discernible character traits in a life that matter, and these traits can be sorted out and embraced.*
>
> BEN CAMPBELL JOHNSON

Wearing his white starched kurta, dohti, and cap (traditional attire worn by male Hindus in the Indian subcontinent), the disciplined, upright image of my paternal grandfather is etched into my earliest memory. I called him Babba. Each morning for him broke in silence and continued with breathing exercises and Sacred Thread yoga. Only then would he rise from his bed and dress in white from head to foot. Every evening upon returning from work, he would bring something for me and my brother, such as a cookie or a bar of chocolate, and many times he would take me out to the food carts for *golgappa chaat*, delicious Indian street food consisting of a small piece of thin bread shell filled with spicy flavorful water. Whenever there was a carnival on Saturdays *(Shanibazaar)*, Babba would give me money.

Thinking back, I realize that none of my grandparents or my parents ever talked about hardship in the presence of us children. There were no complaints from them or tales about how difficult life was. My grandfather was a leader in India, a

barrister who fought for freedom from British rule. He and
Dadiji married at a young age and had eight children, six of
whom lived to adulthood. No suffering, no hardship? Surely
there was, for this is a part of all human life, but it was not
dwelt upon in our household.

In 1942 my grandfather spent a year in jail with other
freedom fighters. Gandhi had said, "Get yourself arrested non-
violently. Fill up the jails and break the British government's
will to rule India." My grandfather and all the freedom fighters
were released in 1943 under an agreement with the British
government and welcomed home as heroes. The people who
had fought for the principles of Mahatma Gandhi and Jawa-
harlal Nehru, the first prime minister of free India, and the
others in the Indian leadership, were representatives of continuing that work in their communities. In 1947 my grandfather
was appointed by the prince of a state called Gwalior as the
minister for health and education. After independence, the
same people continued that work at a global level. My grandfather was appointed National Vice President of the Indian
Cooperative Union, attending meetings of the International
Cooperative Union in Prague, Czechoslovakia. He also traveled
for this work to Berlin, Canada, and Russia. That trip to
Czechoslovakia was when he took me to London to be with my
parents, who were completing their medical specialization
training.

I had no knowledge of all this when my Babba was living. I
only knew he was proud that he had fought with and knew
Gandhi and Nehru, that he was a prominent leader who was
part of the Indian fight for independence for which he had
gone to jail. Instead of sharing details of his work, Babba gave
me experiences that extended and enriched my education
when I was studying geography and history as a preteen. When
I was twelve, for instance, he took me to see the Supreme Court

in session in Delhi. We also visited the 16<sup>th</sup> century Red Fort there for the sound and light show.

Once on a trip to the medieval Qutab Minar in Delhi, Babba told me I could order anything I wanted from the menu at the restaurant. My family, pure vegetarians, had never restricted me from eating non-vegetarian food, but when he said *anything,* I knew he meant it. I ordered a hamburger. During those years I was reading the Archie and Jughead comics. I always wanted to try hamburger and pizza because that's what they ate. Babba never said a thing. That showed tolerance. Besides, my curiosity was satisfied and I didn't crave such food again.

Another recollection of my grandfather's patience and tolerance, also from my preteen years, stands out sharply among others. The whole family was preparing for my aunt's wedding. Everyone had an important task, and mine was to look after my baby brother and keep him out of the workers' way. I decided to cook a special dish to share with him. As I carried the hot food to the serving table, it became more searing by the second. Unable to walk any further without burning my hands, I put it down on one of the metal-frame chairs that had been woven expressly for the wedding with new plastic thread. To my chagrin, the brand-new weaving immediately melted. Standing nearby, Babba calmly said, "That's okay, we'll take care of it." The chair was rewoven in time for the wedding, but at an extra expense. I know now that my grandfather struggled through hard financial times, but back then I wasn't aware of it in the least. Instead of becoming exasperated about the loss, Babba chose to support me and to treat me with understanding.

In his measured and uncomplaining way, Babba would take a morning and evening walk every day. When I was sixteen and started medical school in Goa, he walked with me to the bus stand in the mornings. At the end of the day, he lit a lamp and

the whole family would pray together. Typically, before
entering the prayer area, everyone was to have showered. One
day I had come home late, very tired and irritable, complaining
that I did not want to shower. Babba said, "When your mind
tells you to eat or not to eat, you shouldn't eat, but when your
mind tells you to pray or not to pray you should always pray."
So, I went and showered before joining in the prayers.

After that day, I began to read from our holy book, the
*Ramayana*, which had belonged to Dadiji. In the years after my
Grandmother Dadiji had passed away, Babba would spend
three weeks at a time with us in Goa in our three-room apartment. In our prayer room, where he would sleep, there was a
cupboard built into the wall, a few deities, and a lamp. He'd sit
cross legged in yoga position on his bed. I would sit in a chair
and hold Dadiji's *Ramayana* in my lap. It is a book written in
stanzas, with big print and a few pictures. It's a mythology story
of Lord Ram, about living life. It's the journey of a prince and
his wife and how he is banished from the kingdom to the forest,
triumphing over evil by doing the right things.

These evenings became a tradition of me talking about
what I had read and my grandfather explaining the scriptures
to me after the prayers. Babba would explain how it applied in
today's life. He shared with me words from the scriptures that
he repeated when worried or anxious, a plea to God which says
in Sanskrit:

'दीन दयाल बिरिदु संभारी, हरहु नाथ मम संकट भारी: | |

*Oh, Compassionate One, you already know what I am feeling.
Please take away my fear.*

In this way, night after night, we read the whole book
together. When something ominous happened in the book,
Babba would say "Let's read the next stanza. Let's not end on
anything that is not positive or happy." I practice that even
today. At least once a day for thirty to forty minutes, I read
something spiritual, looking for the positive message.

Three years ago, with both my parents, I again studied the *Ramayana*, which was available as a television series. My Dad would sit with his eyes closed, facing the TV, listening. Both he and my mother have this book memorized. Tears flowed down his cheeks, he was so moved by the beauty of the message and the poetry written in Hindi and Sanskrit. I would hit pause, listen to him reflect on it aloud, then play it some more. It's the same way I read it with my grandfather.

Consciously and unconsciously, I find myself replaying these memories. As I reflect from the current season of my life, it is apparent now to see how much influence my grandparents and parents have had on who I am today. They each have had such a deep impact on how I relate to others as a mother, sibling, physician, educator, leader, colleague, and friend. Their welcoming natures, authentic care, empathetic listening, and balance between flexibility and discipline continue to be my teachers and to guide me as I choose how to show up each day. They give me belonging! Did they know how much they were teaching me?

*Suddenly all my ancestors are behind me. Be still, they say. Watch and listen. You are the result of the love of thousands.*

LINDA HOGAN

# 3 CONNECTING THE DOTS

*Being deeply loved by someone gives you strength, while loving someone deeply gives you courage.*

LAO TZU

MY LIFE HAS GIVEN me the opportunity to live in many different cultures, while allowing me and requiring me to hold onto my own culture. I think not only about belonging but belonging to whom, to what, and at what cost? To answer those questions—to be able to live in this world with no geographic boundaries whether that's due to travel, technology, or social media—it is so important to be mindful of your own ancestral culture and the culture in which you are immersed. My journey goes from India to England to Saudi Arabia to New York to Tennessee. The people in my life are of different cultures and communities and I celebrate that fact.

There are certain parts of our life we celebrate and other parts we are simply grateful for. The early years of motherhood is a season of my life I am grateful for.

## Becoming a Mother

I was in my early twenties and practically a child myself when my daughter was born. In our Indian culture, pregnancies were not public events. A woman was expected to go about her days silently and to pray that everything would go well. My prayers centered on having a healthy baby. I remember the pregnancy itself being pleasant enough. I had the pleasure of my mother's frequent company, as my parents had also moved to Saudi Arabia around the same time for my father's work. I had strong cravings for Perrier water and oranges, along with an equally strong aversion to coffee and tea. I had no baby showers; it was considered a bad omen to celebrate before the baby is born.

We didn't know she'd be a girl. But once she arrived, there were no doubts about the baby's name. She would have a Russian name, Natasha, which was to have been my name. Instead of Natasha, I received the uncommon name Mukta, which means "pearl." This was due to my grandfather's frequent travel to Russia, combined with the political arena in that part of the world—the risk of having a granddaughter with a Russian name was too high. Having a granddaughter with a Russian name would cause suspicion and wasn't worth the risk of losing the trust he'd built as a peace-making government representative.

Mummy surprised me by sewing a receiving gown for Natasha to wear when we brought her home from the hospital. I had seen the perfect newborn dress in a store window. It was a beautiful light pink. I asked my mom to please pick up the dress. Instead she actually stitched a new dress at home with same color fabric and the same lace. My mother wove the threads of her generational love into this gift for me and my daughter. It was gorgeous.

From the hospital, we went to my mother's apartment first instead of to mine. She had a bassinet in her bedroom for the times she'd be caring for her grandchild. It was June and the sun had already set. Everyone else had left the room. I stared down at Natasha in the bassinet, stroking her hair. "I'm your mummy, I'm your mummy." I stood there smiling to myself and crying. A mix of fear, relief, and happiness washed over me, and I collapsed into incontrollable sobbing. After that release, I peered closely into Natasha's face and smiled. She smiled back at me with her tiny mouth, and that was our first encounter as mother and daughter. It was an encounter of souls.

I was an immature and possessive mother. I kept a vital-signs chart with her temperature, pulse rate, respiration rate, intake and output. I would wake her at random to make sure she was breathing. If she made digestive sounds, I was there to measure her output. I did things I knew how to do, but there is no book in the world that truly prepares you for motherhood. When she slept, her eyes rolled back. I didn't know that babies' eyes did that, and I was convinced she was having seizures.

One day I thought it would be okay if I took a quick shower. Wrong! I burst out of the bathroom when I heard her screaming. There she lay in her crib, red in the face. She had caught hold of her own hair, which covered her head in copious amounts. The harder she pulled, the louder she screamed. I broke out into a smile amidst my fears. From then on, no showers for me without another responsible adult present!

The first time I took the baby to India on my own was to visit my family members. Natasha was about twelve months old, and she traveled in my lap holding fast to her bottle. It was a long, arduous trip and I eventually dozed off. I was startled awake to the sight of the poor man sitting next to us, baby spit-up dripping from his sleeve. Are these examples of inept parenting? Perhaps not, but looking back at these mishaps due to inexperience is a humbling experience.

### Becoming a Mother Who Is Also a Physician

Leaving India after completion of medical school, I felt called to study obstetrics and gynecology. I initiated this training between London and Saudi Arabia, in new countries, new cultures, and new training and care environments. (Medical education internationally—then and now—is complicated: the short version is that reciprocal training credit was applicable in some countries and institutions.) Having my parents in Saudi Arabia was crucial for the help I needed to balance both parenting and my work.

I sort of just plunged in and took the risk. When I found out I was pregnant with Natasha, I was fresh into my busy schedule. In fact, I was absolutely in denial. I was under a lot of stress, thinking that's why I had missed a period. And there I was in the field of obstetrics!

My students today often ask me whether or when to get pregnant, worried about financial or time issues or having a support system. I say you have to be open to the fact that it's a blessing to have children and that support will come. There's never a time in life when it's the perfect time to have children. My first child was a surprise and my second one was planned. Both are gifts. Life has a way of giving us what we need. We have to be open to our needs and our realities—whether that is making sacrifices like downsizing or putting your career on hold for a little while. Make those decisions and celebrate what you have at the time, so that you do not have regrets in the future. It's okay to follow your gut and let life happen. My wisdom in this is purely through hindsight.

Both my children were born at the same hospital where I was working. After Natasha was born, I successfully completed my British medical exam. Three years later, in March 1989, ultrasounds clearly showed that my second child was a breech baby. Vigorous kicks at all hours of the day and night were painful evidence that my tiny baby was cramped and uncomfortable in confinement. The surprise came at the moment of birth. All along, we thought that he was a girl! The ultrasound had kept that detail well hidden. My physician exclaimed, "This little boy tricked me!" Nikhil, or Nik as he is known, has been on the move ever since.

Nik was one year old and Natasha was four (and I was twenty-seven) when the Gulf War broke out in 1990. As their father settled into his medical residency in the States, I took the children to India for a few months. The plan had been for me to pack up our place in Saudi Arabia, then the children and I would move to New York at Christmas. But that summer the Gulf War really escalated. My parents talked with us, advising us not to go back to Saudi Arabia. Instead we came straight to America. Who knows how things would have turned out if I'd gone back to the Middle East first?

Traveling alone with two small kids was quite hard, but help came from unexpected places. At the airport of Mumbai (earlier known as Bombay), with massive throngs of people, I had to watch the children, turn in the luggage, and fill out our paperwork for immigration. I had no stroller or bassinet, only my arms. Thankfully, Natasha was calm and a good listener. A group of Indian Roman Catholic nuns who were flying to Rome were very kind. The benevolent nuns kindly took charge of my daughter, entertaining her with coloring books while I finished everything until we boarded the plane.

The nuns disembarked in Rome, and I was alone for the next flight to Manhattan. Nik slept awhile on the plane, but when he awoke, he was unwell with a stomach bug. I left Natasha in her seat and carried Nik up and down the aisles begging desperately for diapers. In India we used cloth diapers, but since living in the Middle East and London, I had used disposable diapers. I thought I had brought enough to get to New York City, but my supply of disposable diapers was exhausted. I must have gotten one diaper from a passenger. Looking back, I was not upset or angry; I just took things in stride, happy to be coming to a new place and grateful Nik didn't have a high fever. My stress was not so much of frustration—it was a good stress.

There are no coincidences or chances. I believe that's where surrender comes in, which leads to me the incredible faith that things do work out.

## Landing in Yonkers

My father's brother and his family lived in Poughkeepsie, New York, and my brother, four years younger than me, was in graduate school at Syracuse. Because they were the only close connections we had in America, we settled nearby in Yonkers, New York.

I consider myself blessed to always be around family and caring communities. I left my parents' home only after marriage and even then, my parents were still in my life as I travelled. Moving between London and Saudi Arabia to the USA was the first time I did not have that security. I shared that concern with Naniji during my visit to India with my kids, before I left for the States. In her usual wise way, she reminded me that I'd be living close to my aunt, "Of course you will not be all alone! You will have Chachiji. Chachiji's home is just like your mother's home." How correct she was. As soon as I landed, Chachiji had equipped our small two-bedroom apartment with all the necessities. Their home was home and to this day is home indeed.

Because my children were so young, I was not prepared to get a job right away in America. I stayed home to care for the children while my husband trained and got relicensed. Medical residencies from foreign countries are not recognized in the

United States—we have to do training all over again to qualify for a license to practice medicine in the US.

In Yonkers, I was glued to the TV quite a lot. My parents and my youngest brother were still in Saudi Arabia and the Gulf War was still underway. Television wasn't part of growing up. I never had access to TV until I was twenty-one. It was also the time of the Anita Hill and Clarence Thomas hearings, with the vivid description of events. I remember thinking, "Oh my God, this really happens?" I had watched a few episodes of Falcon Crest and Dynasty in London and in Saudi Arabia, which showed nothing but these large vineyards, tall buildings, and really rich, sophisticated people. While my intelligent brain told me that America is not always like that, my fantasy brain made me think that's what I would see. Instead, for example, I was told to be careful when walking in the Bronx. It was hard and in many ways shocking to see "the hood" (as I was exposed to the terminology) and the many homeless people in New York.

When we moved to Yonkers, Natasha was not quite old enough for kindergarten as required by the schools in America. What to do? My daughter was a curious child, forever asking questions. She needed more to stimulate her active, inquisitive brain. I located a music school, one that used the Suzuki method, on the easy bus route in front of our apartment. This was to be the beginning of a new season in her life. One day as we were in class, a young East Asian girl sat nearby with her mother. The mother introduced herself and her daughter, and we embarked on a pleasant get-acquainted conversation. The next time we were in class together, she brought information about a school program for early and rapid learners. Not only did she help fill out the forms, she even took me to the school to submit them. It was the beginning of a lifelong friendship for the girls, as well as for us mothers.

After three years living in Yonkers, we moved to another

cultural extreme. In the American medical education system, international medical graduates (IMGs) can qualify for a J-1 Visa waiver[1] by working in underserved rural and inner-city areas of the United States, and that took us to rural Dayton, Tennessee.

On my daughter's first medical check-up with a pediatrician in Chattanooga, my son was all over the place—up and down, up and down, asking questions and interrupting. The doctor, not knowing that I was a physician, could not help but follow my busy son's movements and queried whether he had been tested for attention deficit hyperactivity disorder (ADHD). Returning her question with another question, I asked, "Why would I want to do that?" A bit taken aback, the doctor recovered with, "Just look at him!" Instead I looked directly at her and replied, "No! I am fine, thank you." I never returned to that pediatrician's office, and the startling experience opened my eyes to how flippant and arbitrary we physicians can be and how quickly and thoughtlessly we mislabel a child. And yet I was purely being a mother in that moment, not a physician.

Although I had spent a few years focused on motherhood, I knew I would have to get a job myself and retrain with a third residency. I wasn't thrilled. I loved my life with my children— my adult life has revolved around being a good parent. This maternal instinct fulfills me. I loved having a home full of their friends, baking, cooking, and school activities. My life seemed very full. But I knew it wouldn't be the case long-term. With two children and intentions for their college education, being a two-paycheck family was a given.

In 1994 I worked as an ultrasound technician trainee for a year because I knew it would help me psychologically become okay about leaving the children. In June 1995 I was ready to start my medical training all over again. I would have to retake my qualifying exams and prepare to apply for residency training. Those years away from being a physician and the months as an ultrasound tech gave me time to reflect and think—I didn't want to pursue OBGYN as my career. I would miss the experience of delivering babies, that moment of welcoming a new life. But I wanted what I felt was a more cognitive, intellectual field of internal medicine. I decided to choose the closest teaching hospital, the University of Tennessee at Chattanooga, forty-five miles south of our town.

## Finding Family Next Door

We always knew our neighbors in Goa. That style of living in close proximity was the same in Saudi Arabia and London, and in Yonkers too. But in Dayton, Tennessee, our house had a big yard that created separation between the houses to the left and right. If you didn't attempt to know your neighbors, especially in the dark days of winter, you would be living in isolation. I made a conscious effort to reach out to my neighbors. Within a week of moving there, I made some Indian sweets and left a note with the treats, "I'm excited to be here." I offered to carpool the kids to school. With fruit and cookies in hand, I knocked on my neighbors' doors and they invited me in. That gesture would lead to follow-up phone calls to check on me and get to know me. I met other neighbors in the same way, leading to more reciprocity. I did so not because I wanted anything in return but because it was the right thing to do.

One day there was a knock at the door. I opened it to a married couple who lived close to our home and wanted to welcome us to Dayton—Mr. and Mrs. Morgan, or Tommy and Cherry as we called them. Their daughter had finished nurses' training and moved away. Without children in their home, the two were more than ready to become my children's warm and loving friends. Natasha and Nik grew very close to them. Cherry and Tommy became like godparents. At Christmas they invited the children to a party at their church, but assumed that since we were Hindu, I probably would not want the children to also attend the service. I replied that of course they could stay for the church service! How could my son and daughter value their religious tradition if they did not also take the opportunity to learn about and value other faiths?

With the care extended to our family by these two remarkable individuals, I was able to manage the pressing responsibilities of my residency at the University of Tennessee College of Medicine at Chattanooga and its affiliate hospital. My children were treated like the couple's own children. Cherry and Tommy became willing and able full-time caregivers, picking the kids up at school, feeding them, making sure homework was done, and staying with them when I was away at work. Tommy even fixed things around the house. I would stumble into the kitchen, exhausted from long hospital hours followed by the long commute and presto—the sputtering, leaking faucet leaked no more! We gained not only two lovely companions, but a peace of mind and heart that I could not have imagined possible while balancing a demanding career in a new country.

## A Mother with the Multiple Hats Syndrome

Despite the neighborly support, I was stretched thin with all the hats I wore, striving to perfection in every role: mother, sister, daughter, wife, physician, teacher, friend, colleague, acquaintance, and so on. For seventeen years I left home at six in the morning with both children plus three or four other neighborhood children in the carpool. I'd drop the girls off at the girls' school, the boys at the boys' school, then come to work. After a long day at work, I would pick them up and drop them at whatever after-school practice they had, run to the grocery store, pick up some food for them, come back to the office and work until they finished around seven o'clock, then go home and make sure dinner was ready, clothes were ready, homework was done. And I remember being so angry at myself because I would be screaming all the time, "Come on, let's get to work quickly, get ready!" I'd get up in the morning in a rush and go to bed exhausted completely.

Even though I wanted to create more quality time with my children at the end of each day, I realized I needed to do something to unwind myself first. My best meditation is walking, both the physical act and the time to unwind and reflect. After coming home, especially in summertime, I'd drop everything and tell them, "You do what you need to do, I'm going to go for a walk." I felt so selfish doing that, but when I didn't make time for the walks I felt like I was being a horrible mother and just not a good person. When I did make time for myself and walking, my children and I were then able to enjoy our quality time together before their bedtimes. It became a joke in our house when my children were older; if I were really upset they would say, "Mom, is it walk time?"

It wasn't all bad. On some days, the long commute itself was a great gift. During those years there were no cell phones and no video screens in the car. My kids had a competition about who would sit in the front seat, running to the car to be first. One day when Nik was in third grade, I waited in the droning pick-up line. It was clear that he was in the lead by several car lengths. He jumped in next to me. A moment later Natasha got in the back seat. Breathless and bursting to tell me something, Nik exhaled with, "Mommy, what does the F word mean? Some boys were pointing at that word in a book and laughing. They wouldn't show it to me."

His sister let out an agonized moan, "Ooooh, don't say that word, Nik!"

"Natasha, keep quiet," I said, emphasizing with my eyes to hers in the rear-view mirror. I was simultaneously trying to move away from the cars behind me, wondering how to approach Nik's question, and grieving at the inevitable loss of childhood.

Inspiration hit me. "Nik, let me ask you a question. Where do babies come from?" He promptly answered with confidence, "A girl and a boy get married and they pray to God and God sends them a baby." I held back my tears. What innocence! I wanted to capture that! I knew it would soon be time for me to have the "birds and bees" conversation, but Nik seemed satisfied for the moment. A few weeks later Nik and I had that talk. Except perhaps for book recommendations from friends who are further along on the parenting path, there are just no guidelines to parenting! That day in the car, I was immensely grateful to keep my eyes on the road.

Another afternoon, I heard Natasha talking to her friend who carpooled with us. Her friend was distraught about some mean girls at their middle school. Natasha counseled, "Don't let all that upset you. Just put it out of your mind and think happy thoughts."

In that instant, everything changed for her friend, and for all of us in the car. The remainder of the drive was calm and peaceful. I have since adopted my daughter's example from that day and have made "Happy Thoughts" my mantra.

On any given day, I saw that I could either choose to compartmentalize my life or I could strive to make it as fluid as possible. I can't say "Ok, now I'm a mother, now I'm a wife, now I'm an educator" and shut down the other aspects of myself. During those years I realized there are times for everything. While I don't always have to do everything all at once, whatever I am doing has to be done with more intentionality, even if that's in smaller quantities or for shorter durations.

My son wrote an essay in kindergarten on "My Mother." It included things like "My mother makes cookies. She takes us out. We swing at the park." And the last sentence was, "And also my mother is a doctor."

## Balancing Hats in the Workplace

I changed how I wore my multiple hats at work too. Although most waking hours of our day are spent working, we don't often feel safe in our workplace to speak of anything other than work or to acknowledge that anything is hard outside of work. It really takes courage for a physician (or anyone) to say, "You know what, I need to bring my children here. I'm sorry but I'm drowning in motherhood right now. My child is sick. I can't concentrate on work. I need to go get my child." I wondered how we could create spaces at work where it's safe to be vulnerable and brave.

My daughter was about ten years old when I was a second-year resident. I was working the night call, responsible with another intern. My pager went off at two o'clock in the morning. It was a call from home. I called back and both Natasha and her father picked up. "Mommy where are you? I've had a bad dream." Her father said, "Natasha, go back to sleep. Don't disturb Mommy." He said to me, "She's fine; keep doing what you're doing." We hung up. I knocked on the door of the room where the other resident was sleeping and said, "Look, here's my pager. I'm on call, but I need you to cover my calls." I drove all the way home, only to find her fast asleep, and then I drove back to work again—all those miles!

Phone calls about my children would also come during the day. I started sharing more about my children with my residents and the nurses. I would oftentimes bring my children to sit in the office area while I was doing work. It gave permission to my coworkers to also talk about their children.

When my son was young, it was a chore to get him out of bed. One day I told him, "I have to shout every day and I don't like myself when I do that. If this is the case, I'm going to leave you at the house and I'm going to go off to work." And I did! About an hour later, he woke up and called me, "Mom, where are you?" He was crying. I was crying. I had to tell my colleague, "I need to leave work and go. I've done this, and it took courage, but I have to go back and get him." Nik was never late again. If I hadn't built that relationship with my colleague, I would not have had the courage to say that.

When I was program director and even more so when I was department chair, I gave the faculty and learners permission to let their family lives be part of their work life. I would say, "It's okay if you want to bring your kids to work if you have an hour or two when you need to finish up something. This is part of our life; we don't have to separate it." We had boundaries, of course, but brave spaces need to be both open and bounded. Having our children there occasionally built a community where colleagues were suddenly there for each other in both personal and professional ways.

Around this time, several of my residents were mothers with newborns, struggling with the overwhelm. That led us to establish an informal support network we called "Mommies in Medicine" that was open to medical students, residents, attendings, private practice physicians, staff, and physicians' wives. It lasted only a few years, but served those new mothers well. It led to changes such as ensuring that the hospital's onsite daycare center had room for babies of the residents, so the new mothers could easily drop in.

MY PARENTING WAS A LIVED EXPERIENCE. Those times were so meaningful. I'm grateful that my children were able to adjust to how often I was an inefficient and inexperienced mom. I am also happy they saw me at work in my physician-leader role. Those were pivotal years of growth for me where I realized I can't be a doctor without being a mother, and I can't be a mother without being a doctor. Both roles are integrated. I can't separate the two, and perhaps most importantly, I still don't want to.

As my role of a physician wearing multiple hats expanded further into American health care, the question of "Who am I?" required that I keep exploring to whom and where I belonged —and to continue assessing the cost.

———

*You are only free when you realize you belong to no place—*
*you belong to every place—no place at all. The price is*
*high. The reward is great.*

MAYA ANGELOU

# PART 2

# WHERE DO I BELONG?

*The pain of the world is a cry for belonging.*

JOHN A. POWELL

# 4 MEETING POINT

*If we just worry about the big picture, we are powerless. So*
*my secret is to start right away doing whatever little*
*work I can do. I try to give joy to one person in the*
*morning, and remove the suffering of one person in the*
*afternoon. If you and your friends do not despise the*
*small work, a million people will remove a lot of*
*suffering.*

SISTER CHAN KHONG

DURING MY INTERN YEAR, the first of the three-year
medical residency, I was required to rotate for a month at a time
through various subspecialties. On my cardiology rotation, I
was offered the opportunity to obtain cardiology training under
the direction of a great faculty teacher. Two weeks into my rotation, on a busy day, we were called stat to see a young patient in
her thirties who was unstable with an irregular heart rhythm.
The best management to stabilize her was to externally
cardiovert her, a procedure which restores a normal heart

rhythm in people with certain types of abnormal heartbeats. This is usually done by sending electric shocks to the heart through electrodes placed on the chest.

As our team—my faculty member, a senior resident, and I —entered her room, we saw this young woman staring all around at the commotion caused by nurses and technicians, one placing electrodes on her chest, the other hooking her up to a monitor. All this was going on as one nurse called out orders to another nurse at the door. As we came in, the faculty member quickly introduced himself and began rapidly evaluating the scared young lady while simultaneously placing his stethoscope on her chest to auscultate her heart sounds, his other hand on her radial pulse. Both the faculty physician and the resident knew all the right questions to ask. As the intern, I just stood by their side, unsure of my role.

We followed behind her as she was rushed to the cardiac procedure room with monitors beeping. Her blood pressure was dropping. The rapid response team rushed to perform resuscitative measures. In the procedure room, the faculty shouted out orders to the prepared team standing ready to perform the procedure. The young lady looked on, eyes wide open, when our eyes met. I felt so inadequate and at a loss of how to be useful. I, too, wanted to help. On an impulse I took her hand and felt hers gripping mine in return. Our eyes met again briefly before the sedation was effective. I felt her hand go limp in mine when she was under full sedation effect, but I held on. It made me feel like I was doing something to help.

The procedure was successful, and our patient was sent in a stable condition to the recovery room. The faculty, resident, and I continued our patient rounds. After the end of rounds, we returned to see her. As my faculty mentor started explaining the outcomes, she interrupted him. Her eyes locked with mine as she spoke, "I want to thank that doctor there. She really helped me. She made me feel comfortable by holding my hand." Her response caught me by surprise, which I am sure my face gave away; it also embarrassed me a bit to be complimented in front of my attending and resident. The resident responded with something like, "Yeah she's a good one." I was truly grateful for the patient's affirmation because I thought I had not contributed anything.

## Technology and Touch

If asked to think of one word to describe our world today, we would not be wrong in choosing *change*. The world around us has seen significant changes. Similarly, the world of medicine has also changed. The art of practice and the teaching of medicine has changed. Probably the most noticeable is the advance in technology and its use in almost every field of medicine. We all hold our smart devices, our "peripheral brains" as I call them, in our palm. They allow us easy access to point-of-care knowledge and resources of every specialty. And we physicians are all getting savvier with the use of these smart devices in our palms.

Having my own personal pager was a unique experience for me during my training in the USA, so very different than the personal knock on the call-room by an assistant or the overhead pages by the operators that I was accustomed to in my education and training in India, Saudi Arabia, and London. By 1995 I carried not only my personal pager but a personal flip phone, and then a few years later a smart Palm Pilot, followed by a Blackberry. Just seven years ago I graduated at my children's insistence to an iPhone. At first I felt important, and the world wide web was within my easy reach. I would often find myself distracted or eager to pull out my beeping phone from my white coat pocket to check the source of the message I received. Technology is addictive indeed.

*Where do technology and human touch intersect? How do we*

*discern a balance between the two?* On a typical day as physicians, we make our appointed rounds with pagers or smartphones always attached. These tools of insistent alarm beep intermittently without regard to our train of thought. They interrupt our mental preparation, abort our task list, change the direction of our footsteps, and detour inner commentary. Multitasking, always multitasking, and at what price?

Often when we receive a call from the emergency room to admit a patient, the first thing we do is to switch on and log into the computer, where we will hopefully access essential information from the emergency room doctor's intake. A flurry of exchanges follows—both verbal and electronic—directing the emergency room to initiate appropriate tests, monitoring progress reports, scrutinizing test results, and arriving at a diagnosis before even setting eyes on the patient or giving a reassuring touch to a trembling hand.

I too am guilty. Do I know what brought the patient to the hospital before making decisions to apply a course of treatment? I found myself engaging iPads, computers, and other devices constantly, while subconsciously and even consciously I felt something nudging me, saying that I was not listening as I should or as I taught the students and residents. "Be present for the patient, listen deeply," I would share with them. When these nudges became more than subtle, they were hard to brush aside.

*Shouldn't I be employing my hands to make real-time contact with the patient as well, rather than checking the messages or searching the internet?* Somehow the excuses or rationalization that I was searching information related to the patient did not feel justified or authentic. I knew and realized that technology must be complemented with *touch*. Both are powerful tools, both need to be used appropriately, and neither should be used exclusively. Deep down I knew and believed, and I had personally experienced, that nothing can take the place of human touch and the corresponding relationship-centered care.

## The Power of Our Palms

I wonder at times if we as physicians realize the power of our "palms." In my training days in the early 1980s, I remember the security of bookshelves filled with the classic textbooks of medicine, either in my mentors' offices or in the university's friendly library. I remember thumbing through *Gray's Anatomy*, the bible of medicine, obtaining information. Today, while I still enjoy the smell and feel of a book and the joy of underlining the important information, or making notes to self on the sidebar, it is definitely easier, quicker, and more convenient to just google the information on my iPhone or iPad.

However, I must remind myself that just as I use my iPhone in my palm to decipher a complex acid base balance or a blood gas of a sick patient in the intensive care unit, I must remember to also use my palms to soothe that patient's feverish brow, to hold their hands, to listen to my patient, to examine my patient, and learn from their clinical findings. Just as I use my palm to try to understand the constellation of signs and symptoms of my clinic patient that does not follow the traditional differential diagnosis pattern, I should also remember to use my palms to comfort the patient, reassure them and their family. Just as I use my palm to text my colleague to communicate with them or, to virtually and instantaneously share information, or to discuss common patient management problems, I should also remember to use my palm to extend my hand in thanks, to comfort each other in times of need and sorrow and to share our joy and happiness.

Let us remember to extend our palms to all our patients and colleagues irrespective of their rank, their race, their gender, or their ethnic background. Both our palms and the devices held in our palm are vital to the practice of medicine. They complement each other.

Though technology has contributed to advancing medicine by leaps and bounds, there are certain aspects of medical care that cannot be digitized or put into technology. May we remain mindful that compassion, clinical judgment, connecting with patients, and humanism cannot be digitized.

## Handmade

The post-procedure visit was not the last encounter with that cardiology patient. A week hence, I asked my faculty if he had seen our patient for her follow-up appointment in his office. I was pleased to find that she had improved. A couple of weeks later, an envelope arrived at my department addressed to me. Inside was a beautiful homemade card, a painting of two holding hands. Inside was a note thanking me for holding her hand at a very difficult time. Not recognizing the name right away, it took me a moment to realize who had sent it. A warm feeling washed over me, and I smiled at knowing she had remembered my gesture that I thought was insignificant. I was not inadequate—an affirmation again.

I had not met this woman before, and I was not her physician, but she had made the time and effort to look me up. I received permission to find her phone number and to make a response. I asked how she was feeling and thanked her for her kind gesture, complimenting her artistic talents. I shared with her how meaningful her card was to me, especially as an intern in training.

With this patient I certainly learned about cardiology, and, in the process, I absorbed so much more about empathy-based care: You may not know what to do to cure the patient, but your heartfelt care will go a very long way.

I met that kind patient in 1995, and the experience has never left me. For many years afterward, her special Christmas cards arrived, all of which touched my heart and made me grateful and glad.

*Life is short, and we do not have much time to gladden the hearts of those who make the journey with us. So be swift to love and make haste to be kind.*

HENRI FREDERIC AMIEL

## 5 THE GIFT

*Never worry about numbers. Help one person at a time, and*
*always start with the person nearest you.*

MOTHER TERESA OF CALCUTTA

RESIDENCY TRAINING INCLUDED CARING for patients at
the hospital's health clinic for the community. My first patient
group included a lady in her sixties who had come to the clinic
for a follow-up visit. When I met her, she was sitting down, her
stockinged legs with sensible laced shoes angled to the side.
Wearing a modest floral skirt with a lace ruffled blouse, hair in
a tight bun, my patient appeared to be polished, composed, and
well-educated. She had no serious health-related problems, but
did present some age-related arthritis along with slightly
elevated blood pressure and cholesterol levels. After taking her
full detailed information, I found nothing out of the ordinary
and said I would not need to see her for another six months.

Four weeks later, it was a surprise to see the patient's name
back on my clinic list. I thought of possible reasons: Had I not
communicated well enough? Had she in some way expressed a

concern that I did not address? Perhaps she needed more information on her blood work. "No," she assured me, "I feel fine, but I wanted to be sure."

The next month for a follow-up appointment, she returned, calm and elegant as before. Taking pause, I decided to spend some moments with her in casual conversation. I asked her about her family, how long she had lived in Chattanooga. Her eyes lit up as she spoke of her grandchildren in Florida. Here in Chattanooga, she looked forward to going to church each week, and I had the sense that attending there was her single regular outing. She asked me about my family, being cautious and polite as if unsure whether her inquiry was appropriate. Being a proud mother, I did not hesitate to share stories about my children. She listened and nodded and smiled when I shared their antics. When I described my travels, her thoughtful questions indicated her knowledge and familiarity with the world's current events. Time passed as we chatted. The comfortable conversation and connection we made that day shaped our ongoing relationship.

Thereafter, for two and a half years, I saw her for follow-up visits at the clinic every four to six weeks. She was punctual and never missed an appointment. As our social conversations continued, she always wanted to know more about me than she shared of herself. During my final year of training, just before graduation, when I started to prepare her for care from a new physician, the lady asked for a photograph of myself. I laughed and said lightly, "Now, why would you want a picture of me?" She came back to the clinic twice after her request, but then she missed two appointments.

Becoming concerned, I called her. "How are you? Are you okay? We have missed you at the clinic." Her response was poised but reserved. She shared that she was fine, she had all her medications, and yes, she was in town and not traveling. I grew more curious about why she was missing her appointments. After further gentle probing, she said, "I'm sorry if I disappointed you. Since you didn't give me a picture, I thought I had done something to offend you." Not what I had expected! Obviously, I had failed to give her request the attention it deserved. Inviting her to come back to the clinic, I apologized for not taking her seriously and gave her a small passport-sized photo I had recently taken for my license application.

At the end of June, I informed her that it was my last month of training and that I would be handing over her care to another resident. She responded, "I have been thinking I will move to Florida to be near my daughter and grandchildren. My daughter has been asking me to for a while." Secretly I was happy that she was moving closer to her family, but also sad that I would not see her again.

This last visit was one filled with the unspoken knowledge and sense of an end. We made small talk initially. She thanked me for being her doctor. I thanked her for giving me that privilege, and we wished each other well. I made sure she had the medications she needed and said I would transfer her records as soon as she found a primary care physician in Florida. We exchanged hugs and parted.

## Being Seen, Being Known

About three weeks later, I took a phone call from her in clinic. "You know, I'm going to Florida and thought I would stop by and see you before leaving." Shortly after, my patient quietly walked in. Tucked under her arm was a flat package measuring about twelve by sixteen inches. It was a portrait of me that she had rendered in watercolors from that tiny photograph. What a humbling experience! I thought I knew her, but I really didn't. I hadn't known she was a painter. This artist clearly spoke through her internalized impressions brought to life on paper.

*What if I'd realized that quality of hers earlier on?* This gift of her heart reminded me that communication is the most important attribute in health care.

*Why did she give me this wonderful gift created by her own hands?* Frankly, at that time I felt elated, proud, even boastful. However, years later I am humbled and sad. Sad that I did not express enough gratitude. We stayed in touch for a few months after she left, but as time passed the communication ceased. True, she was a reserved and private lady, but neither did I make more attempts to know more about her Florida family or keep in touch with them. Her painting still hangs in my office. I often ponder the what ifs. The guilt, though lessened, is a continued reminder to not repeat similar missed opportunities.

In 1995 we were not required to carry the demanding, distracting mobile devices 24/7 that often prevent us today from engaging our patients with more presence. We were only distracted if the pager went off. I can't blame my lack of human connection on digital devices. It was my own lack of maturity, or of curiosity, back then. I hadn't known this patient to a significant degree except as she presented herself physically. She, however, knew me on a deeper level.

This fine individual prodded me to think about how every person has a story. In a favorable setting, attended with care, intentionality, and patience, the story of the one in front of us can be offered and received. Without a warm environment of encouraging expectation, we may never truly communicate.

———

*The universe is made of stories, not atoms.*

MURIEL RUKEYSER

# 6 THE LEARNING CURVE

*When care is our first concern, cure can be received as a gift.*
*Often, we are not able to cure, but we are always able to*
*care. To care is to be human.*

HENRI J. M. NOUWEN

EARLY IN MY third year of residency training, a young lady came into the clinic who made a lasting impression on me. Her husband had recently left her in every sense of the word. Without him she was alone and afraid, but with him she had contracted a communicable disease. She tested positive for HIV, a virus causing infection that attacks the immune system, which is our body's natural defense against illness.

Because she had sought out medical assistance and we had been able to identify her physical condition in the early stages, I declared with confidence how now, with improved treatment options, she would have the opportunity to live a near-normal life. The patient's abject response was puzzling. She looked down, was quiet for a few minutes, then broke into a lament of, "Why me? What have I done to deserve this? Why am I being punished? Why, why, why?" A cloud of terrible guilt hung over her, obstructing any thoughts of participation in her own care.

I felt a flash of annoyance as she continued to vacillate and complain about her awful predicament. HIV treatment had made great strides; successful suppression of the virus in the bloodstream of patients was being celebrated. I wanted her to realize this fact. As her weeping continued, it struck me that this young woman had virtually no family support. She couldn't accept that her disease had prospects of improving because she was convinced her affliction was a penance for misdeeds. My irritation subsided and, seeing more clearly, I was able to redirect her attention toward considering pastoral care through our hospital chaplain.

She was initially a "no show" for her scheduled appointments. Our team followed protocol, calling the patient for the first two no-shows followed by a certified letter. Such standard letters inform patients that they would be dismissed from the clinic if they did not keep their third appointment. A full year later, this patient consented to medical care. We may never know why, but the letter may have been one of the reasons she came back for an appointment. I was simply excited to see her and eager to get her treatment started before she changed her mind again.

Her voice was more upbeat, her head was not down and dejected, and she was making eye-contact with me. It seemed she was taking better care of herself. Smiling, she proceeded to tell me how she was connected to a support group through a church. She thanked me and said she would not have taken interest in her own healing had it not been for my encouragement. I referred her to Chattanooga CARES, a Ryan White Clinic which caters to patients with HIV.

## Wholeness is More Than Roles

Reflecting on this experience from so many years ago, I am aware of the personal regret I felt then and often am reminded of, especially when caring for patients who jeopardize their own care. These are the patients we label as "noncompliant" and "frequent flyers" or "bounce backs." They refuse to get the help they are offered for their addictions or seem unmotivated or unable to follow the recommended lifestyle modifications. Some return to the hospital repeatedly, each time with further damage to their health. If I had been more curious about her reasons or had I not made assumptions, I may have learned more about why people are not involved in their own care.

Physicians are trained to talk to patients about preventative medicine, such as by asking, "Did you have your mammogram?" But spiritual conversation is often prevented and sometimes protected. As health care providers we usually acknowledge the many different spheres of life—social, mental, emotional, and physical. But it's vital to also honor the person's spiritual dimension. The spirit actively generates the "glue" that binds all dimensions of life together.

The young woman who initially refused treatment did so because she viewed her experience of loss through an opaque lens of guilt and punishment. Her spiritual stance led her to make a decision against life. As her physician, I could have served her with spiritual support myself in conjunction with the medical and physical support so that she may have seen how to advance her health instead of mourning it.

*What if I had taken a more spiritual approach myself and explored her vulnerabilities and hesitations, instead of getting frustrated?*

My patient's experience stands as a vivid example of how our outlook influences our health. Any single life event can be perceived as a medium for spiritual change; every event holds promise as an avenue for positive change.

I now understand how critical it is for physicians to consider *all* of what their patients need, not only at the physical level, but also at the spiritual, emotional, and mental levels. Even today I still need to remind myself and continue to hold myself to this core principle in evaluating my practice— remembering to ask about the wholeness of my patients' lives.

As an educator today acknowledging this central premise to my residents, I refer to the response that most of us routinely make to the question, "Who are you?" We answer with the name of a role, such as Student, Mother, Daughter, Physician, Educator, Administrator, Sister, Wife, Aunt, Volunteer, or Technician, and we want to call this role a life. We think that if we knit all these fragmented roles together, the fabric of our mantle will be complete. But no, this isn't what life is about!

As I reflect on what about these roles makes me feel content or fulfilled, I realize it is the *relationships* I have in each role. The relationship is what connects me or touches me deep in the center and creates that warm indescribable feeling. I can't authentically live *with* people by only performing a role or three. Living *with* others would then exist without meaningful relationships or connections. I must live *for* others instead.

Living *for* people means I accept them for who they are, striving to be open to both similarities and differences of any kind. I acknowledge my own feelings about them even if they are negative, without judgment. I strive to build a relationship that invites us to agree to disagree. This to me is the basis of spirituality. When I live for people, I am relating to them based on what matters to their spirits, thereby developing personal and meaningful relationships. This is hard.

## Teamwork Supports Wholeness

I used the chaplain service more readily after this experience. Years later in my role as chair of the department of medicine, I initiated a routine of multidisciplinary rounds for each patient on the teaching teams which met every afternoon. The team included a case manager, pharmacist, physical therapist, legal aid, dietician, assigned chaplain, the patient's nurse, and physician team. Each team member contributed their patient's history from their lens, sharing our view of the patient's needs, our plans, and our concerns in an attempt to be mindful of delivering true patient-centered holistic care.

People bare themselves to physicians in unconditional trust, revealing their physical, mental, emotional, and spiritual states. My team regularly discusses what it means to be called to compassion, "to walk beside" our patients instead of settling for roles as simple data exporters or bearers of important information. Working on a daily basis with a team, I can serve our patients with even more vigor and determination.

I once read that people can see life in one of three ways: Helping, Fixing, or Serving. Those who practice *helping* learn to see life as weak. Others who go about *fixing* people find themselves viewing everyone as broken. It is only when we *serve* that we experience life as whole. My encounter with this particular young patient, and its subsequent learning curve, came with a clarion call that I was meant to serve.

Serving is about spirituality. I strive to serve by helping my patients understand their illness, make them feel better cared for and comforted. Actually, we help each other. Our patients teach us more than the text books. Patients teach us how to cope, to find meaning and purpose in the midst of—and in spite of—illness and suffering. At its center, healing is spiritual. Thus it follows that as we resolve to follow the vocation of healing, my team and I can look for ways to restore healthful whole-ness amid hardship and affliction.

## Spirituality Includes Self Care

The topic of spirituality continues to be researched as an active contributor to well-being and rejuvenation. If we know spiritu-ality is important, why don't we act on it? Could it be true that as health care providers pose spiritual questions to patients, we, too, are in conflict and searching for solutions for our own hearts?

*How in turn can we physicians face our own vulnerabilities instead of avoiding them? Do we burst and shatter from unbearable pain, or collapse into our own version of a black hole?*

Consider the humble tortoise, who carries his own shell, not easily broken. I collect tortoise figurines. The more hand-made they are, the better I like them. I discovered tortoises in our yard when we moved to Tennessee. I think they are such wise and fascinating creatures. A few years ago, I arranged for three of my residents to present their ground-breaking research work at an international conference in Hawaii. I had to jump through a lot of hoops to get the funding. When they came back, the students brought me a gift of a handmade tortoise. They had no idea I loved tortoises.

"Dr. Panda, this reminds us of you. Wise and calm."

I said, "Really? Is that me?"

I kept thinking about that analogy for myself, feeling more vulnerable than wise and calm. I received the tortoise gift around the time I was considering where I belonged in my personal life and professional life. I felt I had been retreating and hiding myself for so long. (I'm going to mix my metaphors for a moment.) I would take off and put on different hats depending on who I was with—my children, my parents, my students, my spouse. Who *was* I at that point? I decided I really needed to get out my shell. The shell protects the shy inner self, just as the hat shades the eyes from harsh sunlight or signals to others what they can expect of us. But if we hide our whole self forever inside the shell, or live a life where we do not honor the many roles we play as humans, we cannot experience wholeness.

The residents' gift gave me a new interest in reflecting upon what these creatures really symbolize. The tortoise has its own inner life and is able to retreat without being harmed. The tortoise, a living being of God, also carries a halo of the divine. Humanity blithely builds its own version of shells, but not with mindfulness or intention for good. Human beings, as if sleep-walking, allow the popular culture and environment to shape their shells, layer upon infinite layer. Our human shells are inflexible. They break in jagged halves, suffocate with terrible weight, or abruptly explode around us.

When we avoid integrating the many roles in our lives, it's like wearing too many hats until the weight of them all obscures our vision and damages our health. These days when I speak with colleagues and other physicians regarding well-being, I refer to what I call the Multiple Hats Syndrome. I show a slide with different images of hats and ask, "Which one is yours?" I say "You diagnose so many syndromes in other people, but you also have to think about diagnosing yourself. That's where self-care starts—by diagnosing yourself." Showing the slide again, I ask them to reflect on how they can integrate the many hats they wear.

A tortoise can't live without its shell, and so by the grace of nature, the outer shell grows as the creature grows inside. We humans must grow in self-awareness. Unlike a tortoise, our emotional shell can go from being protective to unproductive, especially when our needs for belonging and safety go unmet. It was time to face my own vulnerabilities instead of avoiding them.

*I have seen many storms in my life. Most storms have caught me by surprise, so I had to learn very quickly to look further and understand that I am not capable of controlling the weather, to exercise the art of patience and to respect the fury of nature.*

PAULO COELHO

# 7  DIFFERENCES AND DISCRIMINATION

*Give the real you a chance.*

DESMOND TUTU

THE WORD "DISCRIMINATION" was never in my vocabulary until I came to America. In the Middle East and London, I didn't use that word. I grew up in a culture where we were always aware of and often talked about the caste system. I strived to belong from a very young age. I felt this desire for belonging as a sense of wanting to be with people. But I never felt I was being discriminated against.

I only articulated the word "discrimination" when I got to the United States. It was a very harsh word when it first popped into my brain. When I entered the workforce in the US, I felt a lack of general acceptance and a need to prove myself in a different way, beyond proving myself through good work. Only then did "discrimination" come into my mind. As I reflect back, I find it hard to pinpoint and articulate what it was that made me feel a sense of being different. India is not only land of the caste system, but of multiple cultures, religions, languages, food, and attire. When my family moved to Goa from New Delhi (after living in London), we were different because we were from the north, yet that felt normal and accepted.

As soon as I first landed in Yonkers, I received unsolicited advice from former colleagues who had family in New York or had visited. Some warnings were explicit, some subtle, to avoid certain areas. "Do not use the subway. Avoid these stores. Be careful where you go. Keep your belongings close to you. Do not travel alone. Be careful to protect your children, or they may go astray and rebel against the more conservative Indian culture." It was as if the sense of being different was introduced then.

In the neighborhood where I lived, very few people spoke Hindi, the native Indian mother tongue, or wore the native attire of the saree or the traditional loose baggy pants called *salwar* with a long top called a *kameez*. But people were cordial and nice. This was a growing period for me. My children were almost two and four. I wanted to make sure I raised them to be comfortable in the USA but also worried that they not forget their roots and their Indian cultural heritage.

Three years later we moved to Dayton, Tennessee, a small town north of Chattanooga with even fewer Indian families. We were one of three families from India in our five-mile long city. This was the first home we ever owned. The first time we invited some work colleagues to our home in Dayton, I was nervous, scared, and tired. It was really hard enough to follow the norms and etiquette, to make sure that my family was worthy to belong. I went out and bought an ice tea maker and practiced making iced tea because I knew that was something everybody drank in Dayton. In India we drank our tea hot and with milk. I worried. Would our colleagues like the food? Would I serve the right wine and cheese? What should I wear, Indian or Western? I thought I had covered all the possible points to worry about.

The guests were all in the kitchen where I had laid out the dishes in a buffet style. As we gathered around the island, I explained the various dishes, sharing their Indian names and translating the ingredients and the level of spice for the guests. After I finished, one of the female guests who was facing the kitchen window pointed outside, asking, "What's that building?" She was referring to a small shed that stood detached but by the side of our home, basically a big unfinished room.

"That's an outhouse," I said. Outhouse is a word commonly used in India to mean a building used for storage or as an extra room to house workers. Years later I learned the American meaning of outhouse. I am still cringing as I recollect this scene twenty-eight years later. My guests responded with a nod, a strange smile, but no follow-up questions. I'm not sure if they laughed behind my back, but I did get some strange looks that day.

Learning colloquial language has really served me well. I did initially ask for a "torch" when I was examining the eyes of my first patient. Luckily for me, my senior resident was a kind gentleman, so while he laughed, he was also quick to teach me. I am grateful for my ability to laugh at myself. Otherwise my residency training would've been hard. It took me a while to stop using words like dustbin for the trash can, or boot for the trunk of a car, or to stop pronouncing certain medical terms with the emphasis on the wrong syllable. I now have a colloquialism dictionary that I share as I orient the non-US graduates.

These were the easier challenges I faced. It was during my residency program that I became more aware of discrimination against international medical graduates.[1] I remember being warned by another non-US senior resident two years ahead of me to be very mindful because the chief resident, a US graduate, was reviewing our patient notes behind our backs and reporting to the leadership any mistakes he thought were made. A rumor was that the administrative staff was instructed to keep two piles of residency applications that were submitted, one for the US graduates and one for the non-US. I have to be honest; I did not seek to validate or confirm these rumors. The possibility was enough to instill fear and a level of distrust.

When you face discrimination, your heart sinks and breaks. You try to fit in. You doubt yourself. You feel guilty and ask "what's wrong with me?" You feel so guilty you try to improve yourself, but after a while, you realize you're fighting a losing battle. You can build up resilience by taking a big deep breath, trying to not let it affect you. Or you can choose to retaliate— and that's not right for me. I felt lonely as a nonwhite female and as a non-US graduate, an immigrant. In response, I built up an emotional armor-like shell that was very difficult to crack. If only we would allow our hearts to crack open to let the light in, as Leonard Cohen sings. A "broken-open heart" is more malleable and can absorb more than a broken heart.

We become insecure from a toxic culture of being watched or the perception of being watched (both are real), and that insecurity threatens our emotional and psychological safety. This illustrates how the basic need of belonging in Maslow's hierarchy can go unmet. While health care in America is so dependent on talent from all over the globe, the political scenario does not easily value or accept non-US physicians. In fact, international medical graduates and immigrant physicians face discrimination, both at personal and policy levels. The 2017 executive order to ban immigration restricts acceptance of non-US physicians into our medical training programs. This increases our stress and burnout, dismissing (if discussed at all) how we add value with our different cultural experiences and our bilingual or multi-lingual capacity.[2]

Graduate medical education is an emotionally and physically demanding time for all physicians. Minorities in medicine are not only from outside the United States. Black, Latino, and Native American residents experience additional burdens secondary to race/ethnicity. For example, a study reported in *JAMA* in 2018 describes a daily barrage of microaggressions and bias, minority residents tasked as race/ethnicity ambassadors, and challenges negotiating professional and personal identity while seen as "other."[3]

While I, too, can relate to those same challenges, other things now seem less important to me, such as feeling left out of the conversations about baseball or football. I adapted by trying to learn the American culture myself and educate my colleagues about mine. I was determined to not feel like a victim. I decided that I needed to take responsibility to learn, to seek to understand and acknowledge the new customs, to acculturate *and* enculturate, to strive to belong and offer belonging. Life began to improve and, by and large, I could relate to most of my colleagues.

## Believing in Myself

At the end of my residency, it came as a shock when I was asked by the leadership of the department if I wanted to stay on as faculty. I am grateful because this first invitation opened the door to so many opportunities that have led to an amazing journey for me.

More doors opened in the first few months of becoming faculty when I was invited to several important committees in the hospital and the university. It was so flattering. One day on a phone call with my parents in India, I was describing the different work I was involved in. By hearing myself speak aloud, it dawned on me, *I am a minority!* The invitations were because I was a minority. Of course, I was an international medical graduate, but I hadn't specifically thought, *I am a minority.* I was viewed as the minority because I was from India and did not have the same color skin or hair as others. At first, I was a little upset about it, but then I decided, *You know what? I'm going to celebrate it. I'm going to learn so much.*

But did I belong? I soon realized it had been easier to fit in as a resident in training than as faculty. Faculty was a totally different playing field. Discrimination is not always blatant, but is an accumulation of moments like being snubbed by another faculty member or boss, or seeing less qualified colleagues receive choice assignments. The feeling of powerlessness can be overwhelming. I can't quite put my finger on it, but I felt as if we international medical graduates should be indebted for being given a position in which to train and that our color, gender, or nationality made us in some ways inferior.

Sometimes I spoke with other non-US colleagues about this vague sense of discrimination. These were times when I could unload and be true, or when I could actually have a pity party and let myself feel like a victim.We non-US graduates were together and a common humanity joined us. But I also realize, looking back, that we were scared and didn't feel that any unity in numbers could give us some voice.

Being faculty was an uncomfortable place to live and work. However, that sense of discrimination changed with leadership at different levels, where some people very much embraced and celebrated diversity. Fortunately for me this happened relatively early in my faculty role.

I believe in the saying that when life deals you lemons, make lemonade—and not just in one flavor, but in many flavors and whatever color you want. You have the power to choose your response. I decided to accept those invitations to committees with that empowering attitude. And those were such amazing learning opportunities and networking. I was able to connect with people that perhaps I would never have had the opportunity to meet. Moreover, I was being introduced to the concept of medical teaching in a more formal and structured way. I truly enjoyed learning and received positive feedback. Over time, even more doors opened.

## A Fellowship Opportunity

About a year after I joined the faculty, the department chair said, "Mukta, I think you should apply for this fellowship in faculty development at the University of North Carolina in Chapel Hill."

I looked into the fellowship and it sounded really exciting. I would only need to go to Chapel Hill three times a year for four days, while the rest of the coursework experience would be online. The opportunity was a good fit because I would not have to leave my family, and that meant a lot to me. The only thing was, the program was limited to ten fellows from all over the country every year. I told my department chair, "I'd love it, but they take only ten people."

"Why do you think you're not worthy enough? Of course you are! But how will you know if you don't apply?"

His support helped me have the courage to believe in myself. And when I got in, I thought, *Wow, I can do this!*

My fellowship cohort was small and diverse, from varied US and non-US backgrounds. It felt like I had gained a group of kindred spirits with a shared covenant to be the best we could be as physicians, educators, and leaders. Many had similar backgrounds as mine, immigrating to the US after training abroad or having other careers prior to medicine. This gave me courage and some sense of security, and finally the belonging I was craving. I was grateful that these conditions created a safe space in which we could share ideas and experiences. With them I was exposed to larger networks of national organizations and meetings. I was introduced to faculty who were working on addressing acculturation issues in training programs. I got a chance to work with them, presenting work-

shops and co-authoring chapters in manuals for program directors. I was able to find my authentic voice. That fellowship
opened multiple doors, and since then I've remained as faculty
in multiple leadership positions.

I witnessed one of the first blatant examples of discrimination after my fellowship training. Midway through one afternoon clinic session, there was a brief lull in the busy schedule. I
decided to get a cup of tea and invited one of our clinic leaders,
a black woman, to accompany me. We went to the physician
lounge, which was empty at the time. As we were getting the
tea, a male physician who is white walked in and started chat-
ting with us. A few minutes later, in came another older white
physician—a well-respected, long-standing physician in the
community who had been one of my faculty during my residency and was now a peer.

It soon was obvious that he was returning from a high-
stakes meeting that did not end to his expectations. He
started describing this meeting in which he was trying to
mediate negotiations between two groups. It became
apparent that one group was generally made up of people of
color while the other was primarily white. As he expressed
his frustrations, he referred to "Black Sambo." I do not
remember the entire conversation in detail, but I did notice a
pained look on the clinic leader's face as she fled from the
lounge. I ran behind her, shouting her name as she raced
toward the clinic. I caught up with her, touching her arm
from behind, and she turned around. I saw anger, pain, and
tears in her eyes. I asked her what happened. She looked at
me and said, "Did you not hear what he said?" I was ignorant
and said, "No, I did not. Look, I am sorry. Please explain
to me."

"He made racial remarks," she said.

That was enough. I said, "I am so sorry. What are we going
to do? What if you talk to him and let him know how you feel?"

"No! No!" she was quick to respond. "He is powerful. I will lose my job. No, please, let's be quiet."

"No, we can all go," I said. "I will ask the other faculty who was there."

"No, he will not do anything. I do not want to cause trouble."

I was sad. "I saw it. I will say something." As we kept talking, I assured her that I would do something and also that I would make sure I would not cause her any harm to the best of my ability.

I was not sure what to do. First, I went to the always-available Google to educate myself on the story of Black Sambo. After reading varying versions of the story and its interpretations, I knew I had to say something. I wanted to go the department leadership, but they were at a meeting out-of-state. I decided to speak to the faculty who had made the remark. I was scared because he was an icon. At the end of the clinic, I was walking back to the hospital when I saw him walking toward me. I stopped him and requested a minute. I remember having to tilt my head to look up into his face.

"I think what you said to the clinic leader today was inappropriate." I could see he was taken aback.

After a brief pause, he said, "That's how I speak. That's how I was brought up."

I do not remember my exact response, but in essence I told him I could not change how he felt, but that his comment was unprofessional, and it was inappropriate to behave like this at work. I remember even telling him that if this did not change, I could not allow him to precept the residents under my direction. Somewhere in the middle of the conversation, he interrupted me, saying that this was how it was.

"Such behavior is not okay now," I said. "You would not want to behave like this in front of your grandchildren either." Then I said thank you and left. I can't name my emotions in that moment, but as I walked to the hospital I had sweaty palms, a racing heartbeat, and a sense of accomplishment mixed with fear. This feeling continued for a few weeks with similar intensity, evoking a physical and visceral response. I shared the encounter with the leadership a few days later. I was listened to, complimented on my initiative to call out the wrong, and invited to return if the issue recurred.

While it's possible to remain cordial and professional after such a confrontation, which we all did, I don't know if any hard feelings lay tangled beneath the surface.

## Celebrating Who We Are

*Who am I? Where do I belong?* Especially in 2001 after the September 11 terrorist attacks, these questions resurfaced in my mind with more urgency. As a family from India living in Tennessee, we wondered how to handle the fears about non-white people that arose around that time. I always dressed in Indian clothes at formal occasions. I felt overall that "if we are who we are" we would be accepted. But after September 11 we decided to hang an American flag outside our house.

A week or two later, Natasha and a friend who is white were driving home from a high school football game in Chattanooga. Some boys in a Jeep yelled at my daughter, "Traitor, go back home!" She told me about it during our commute that evening, upset but curious how to respond. We decided that whenever there was an opportunity, we would celebrate our heritage and educate people about India.

On "World Day" at school that year, Natasha celebrated India. That's when I began thinking about where we belong and how to show it emphatically to the children, but Natasha showed me. For the talent showcase in her senior year, Natasha choreographed a Bollywood song to perform with her class-mates. They all wore traditional Indian dress that night, which was a moment of real pride and joy for me. To celebrate her, I wore a traditional salwar kameez outfit too.

On a different occasion, Natasha went against her school's protocol. The tradition in that private school was to make your senior presentation independently as your moment to shine. Natasha invited all her community to be part of her presentation as a celebration. To me, it was such a courageous thing for her to do.

Natasha continued to bring people together by applying her passion for dance and compassion for children to her volunteer efforts. One summer in Goa, India, she volunteered at a *Dishaa* school for disabled children (children who are ostracized from Indian society) and choreographed a beautiful dance for them in Hindi about being stars on earth. These children made earthen lamps, which she bought years later to use as center-pieces at her wedding. And then just after her undergraduate college education she conceived of a fundraiser to help build a playground for the young special-needs children, particularly those with autism, at the Siskin Children's Institute in Chattanooga. Original choreographed dances accompanied by her narration of stories from the varying states of India wove her best personal qualities and those of her mother country into a fantastically conceived production. She called her independent creation, *Nashaa, Dancing through India*. For the dance crew, she enlisted a large, ethnically and physically diverse circle of high school and college schoolmates. Not one was a professional dancer, but each girl had great devotion to the project. Natasha's friends spent countless, tireless hours learning new dances of an unfamiliar culture as they rehearsed together for their courageous show at the historic city auditorium.

As soon as the program ended, Natasha came running out to her family in the audience. She was seeking mainly one particular approval. "Did you like it?" After a long moment, the reply, "Yes, but you could have chosen better dancers." The crowd had loved the performance, but she only sought this approval! Her response? "You missed the point. The whole idea was about celebrating differences." Her passion was not deterred. And to this day, children with challenging disabilities are still playing and climbing all over that playground and learning what they can do, one movement at a time.

Natasha continues to dance, a God-given gift which she shares with many. In her words, she dances for her soul! Her innate perceptiveness to recognize and focus on the heart language of people is a glue, a uniting force that sustains our family in so many ways. She shows respect to the elders, the younger, to Americans and non-Americans. In so many ways, she is my teacher.

*HOW DO I believe in myself despite discrimination? And how do we invite others to join in as we celebrate who we are?* To me, it's about reciprocity. Because I've faced not feeling welcome, I go out of my way to make others feel welcome. I now intentionally try to make conversation with people who have ignored me so I can try to break down barriers. I love Gandhi's words, "Nobody can hurt me without my permission." I make a conscious effort to say hello to people. I try to engage in more meaningful conversations. I send birthday greetings to my former students, a small gesture but it's important to remember them because they touched my life in some way.

When I feel someone cares about me as a person, beyond being a medical physician, I want to know more about them. I may tend to gravitate to people who ask me about my family, with honest curiosity to learn more. But I gravitate toward people, period, and this is one way I survive. Finding our common threads makes me feel like I belong, like I want to go above and beyond with a sense of deeper caring.

*In everyone's life at some time our inner fire goes out. It is then burst into flame by an encounter with another human being. We should all be thankful for those people who rekindle the human spirit.*

ALBERT SCHWEITZER

# 8  HOUSE CALLS

*I paint life.*

ROBERT E. RITTENHOUSE

A DIFFERENT QUALITY of conversation often arises with my patients when I see them over the course of many appointments. In an unfolding relationship, we open up and share candid stories of our lives—the mundane joys and significant heartaches, the challenges and celebrations. I am changed by the patients I meet, and sometimes so are my children. One such patient was Rob Rittenhouse, who I met in January 2002.

It was a busy clinic day and nearly 4:30 p.m. when Rob checked in for his first visit. As practicing physicians, we know that when this happens we have to prepare ourselves for our clinic to be extended beyond the normal hours of 5:00 p.m. New patient visits must be detailed and thorough and take more time, even longer in a teaching hospital. As per policy, any new patient is first seen by the resident in training, who takes a detailed history and does a physical exam and then presents the information to the faculty preceptor. Both then see the patient together. Such redundancy is necessary in order to ensure an appropriate diagnostic workup and to role model clinical decision-making for the resident.

After my resident relayed to me the patient's story and reason for his visit, we went into the exam room together. That is when I first met Rob. By then it was 5:15 p.m. and the sky was getting dark. The exam room had no windows and the bright neon tube lights revealed a smiling gentleman sitting on the chair with his wife beside him. I pulled up the stool to face Rob and his wife, Yvonne, with my resident standing by my side. Introducing myself and shaking hands with him and his wife, I proceeded to validate his story and exam findings for myself.

For six months Rob had been bothered by intermittent foot drop and leg weakness. His condition remained undiagnosed and became increasingly annoying, despite having sought treatment from several physicians in the small town of Cleveland, Tennessee. Rob and Yvonne had recently relocated there from Washington state to be closer to her family. In addition, he was having trouble executing fine brush strokes onto his canvases. Rob's complaints were vague, and I knew—putting on my clinician and educator hats—that the possibilities, or differential diagnoses, were vast.

Rob remained calm as he replied to my numerous inquiries. Yvonne stood by his side with a look of concern. While Yvonne was quiet for most of the visit, she often nodded in agreement, occasionally adding a word or sentence to confirm or clarify as Rob told his story. Rob often looked at Yvonne for affirmation. Her strength and her care for her husband was palpable. As I left the exam room after that first visit, Yvonne smiled with a combination of gratitude and anxiety as she held my hand and said thank you.

Over several visits, I learned more about them. Yvonne spoke more readily, asking clarifying questions about our thoughts, taking notes, and marking the appointment dates in her calendar. She shared Rob's love for painting, reading, and playing chess.

Following in the footsteps of Sherlock Holmes (whom Rob admired and compared us with), my resident and I replaced our physician hats with detective hats and embarked on the path of diagnostic testing. Within a few weeks, we had our conclusion. My gut instinct and fears had come true. His diagnosis was Amyotrophic Lateral Sclerosis (ALS), also referred to as Lou Gehrig's disease. ALS has no known cause. The disease kills nerve cells, eventually rendering the person disabled, and leads to fatal complications.

I felt unprepared and unsure how to deliver this news. I was upset with Rob's diagnosis myself. Though my training did teach me the general principles for delivering bad news, when it came to actually doing so, it was hard. I often say that I can never keep a poker face and this is still true today.

It was February 7, the morning before his fifty-fifth birthday, when my resident and I gave Rob the verdict. His wife was with him and so was their pastor. I sat down facing the three of them. I only remember my soft voice having a lot of pauses and ums. I don't exactly recall the words of our conversation that day, but the emotions—both my own and everyone's in the room—are still vivid and poignant.

Rob was well-informed and immediately understood what his diagnosis meant. I was truly taken aback by the strength and composure shown by those three amazing individuals. Yvonne was holding Rob's hands and their pastor had his hand on Rob's shoulder. I find myself tearing up as I write this. I remember the immense gratitude, the calmness and strength in the room, coupled with their lack of anger or fear. I was surprised. I expected more questions. His eyes simply spoke volumes that afternoon but were clear with confidence and peace. It was apparent that Rob and Yvonne shared an unconditional faith, one that I had come to understand and honor through our many conversations. That day I received the gift of a relationship that made it easy for me as a physician to build a partnership with my patient and his family.

Rob was fully aware of the natural course of the disease. ALS cannot be cured and has few treatments to improve the quality of life. With a firm sense of self-worth and spiritual strength derived through faith, Rob elected to remain at home, work in his studio, surrounded by his paints, brushes, and easels. He knew it was a matter of time, over which he had no control. He expressed this sense of surrender with calm wisdom, saying he wanted to live his life to the fullest and to the best of his ability. He also found the courage to state jokingly but with conviction that his only wish was that he would go while he could continue to wipe his own bottom.

By mid-March Rob had continued to weaken and required a wheelchair. He was still able to take care of his basic needs with occasional help, his devoted wife always by his side if needed. I learned more about this man over the next few months by talking with him, his wife, his pastor, and my resident. Rob was an internationally ranked expert chess player as well as an expressive painter. He was also, as alluded to above, an avid fan of Sherlock Holmes. We enjoyed conversation about how my son shared these interests. One day Rob said, "I'd love to meet your son."

I, too, wanted my son to meet the wonderful human being that I saw in Rob's eyes and his wife's eyes. I wanted my son to be part of that. With permission from Yvonne, who was delighted, I decided to pay Rob and Yvonne a visit with my resident and Nik.

## A Most Memorable House Call

It was a hot afternoon at the end of June when I picked up Nik from summer camp and told him today was the day we were visiting Rob.

Rob was sitting upright in his wheelchair when we arrived. He was still able to hold a brush using his left hand as support and was rendering a portrait of his great-niece. After introductions, Nik and Rob went off to have a game of chess. I do not know the conversation they had in those forty-five minutes. They both had a different look on both their faces when they rejoined us. I simply wanted Nik to have a chance to play chess with this chess master. I had nothing else in mind.

Rob seemed hesitant to let us leave, which Yvonne noticed. She invited us to stay for sandwiches. Nik was fairly quiet the rest of the night. The peace, the calm, and the hospitality that both Rob and his wife shared with us that evening were amazing and palpable.

After we ate, Rob gestured toward a watercolor on his living room wall that he'd painted of a Bosnian girl, one who had been resettled with her family through a Christian refugee assistance agency in the Pacific Northwest. The portrait was serene and peaceful, in stark contrast to the young girl's recent experience in her war-torn country.

Rob offered me a gift—my choice among several paintings. "Or," he quipped with a chuckle, "you can look at this one," turning in the opposite direction. "It is interesting, but not very pretty." He called this piece, "The Obnoxious Bird, the Bird from Down Under." The piercingly fierce, reddish glare of this portrait captured my attention. I asked how the painting got its name, and he happily related how the expression in the emu's eye had captivated his imagination while on a photoshoot with his wife at the Woodland Park Zoo in Seattle. Gazing at this enormous, gray, and ungainly bird, the emu seemed to be saying, "Even though I am not the prettiest of birds, I am proud of who I am."

I looked into the eye of the painted emu and felt as though I was seeing straight into Rob's eyes the day he learned of his diagnosis. It was a face that said with an air of unblinking confidence, "I am proud. I will not give up. I will fight." That was the true spirit of Rob Rittenhouse.

As we walked to the door to leave, Yvonne handed me a brown paper bag full of books about Sherlock Holmes and chess. At first, I refused, "Oh we can't accept. We will only borrow them." Rob laughed and said, "You'll be borrowing them a long time."

Nik took the books and I carried "The Obnoxious Bird" in my hands. Rob wished Nik all the best. I had a profound sense that this was my last meeting with Rob. Nik was silent on the drive home, sitting in the back seat instead of scrambling to sit up front as usual. I was tearful, talking randomly about what a wonderful couple they were, thanking Nik for coming with me. In a quiet voice, he said, "Thank you, Mom, for bringing me along."

That night around the dinner table, Nik told Natasha about our day. Days later she quietly gave Nik a copy of the book, *Tuesdays with Morrie*. She could tell his heart had been opened to a new path. Although Nik and Natasha shared the common sibling rivalry growing up, the deep care, love, and friendship they felt for each other deep down has blossomed in their adulthood. It is beautiful to watch. As their mother, I am grateful.

## Orientation Day

I took Rob's painting to work the next day, placing it on a chair in my office. I wanted to share my visit and show the painting to the clinic nurses and staff and, of course, my resident. He had left earlier than Nik and I.

The end of June is when our senior residents graduate after three years of training and are eligible to be certified by the internal medicine boards and to practice independently. This is also the time we welcome a new class of residents starting year-one of residency training. I was charged with orienting the new residents to the clinics, the process, and their goals and expectations. I had a formal presentation prepared. My heart was still full of emotions about visiting Rob and Yvonne the day before, my mind occupied with thoughts of our meeting.

On an impulse, I said to the clinic nurse, "I don't think I need a PowerPoint today. I'm going to do something different."

I shortened my detailed presentation and brought in the painting. I held it in front of the residents and staff and asked them to share what they saw. They responded to the obvious: a bird, an ostrich, an emu.

"Let me tell you what I see," I told them. "I see a wonderful human being, a gentleman, who has taught me lessons that are not found in the textbooks of medicine." I then described Rob's health situation and my journey with Rob and Yvonne. I invited them—and challenged them—to strive to establish relationships with their patients like I had with Rob and Yvonne. I said it was not only a suggestion but something I really hoped for them. "These relationships will teach you about life, courage, resilience, and the strength to face suffering and live with grace even in hopeless situations."

I was very pensive after the orientation session, but felt full and grateful. I called Yvonne, wanting to share what I had done and offer gratitude. My call went to voicemail. It was Wednesday, the day Rob still tried to attend church if he felt strong enough. Presuming that's where they were and certain Yvonne would get back to me, I did not call again. She did not call back on Thursday either. Feeling worried, I called Friday morning.

A nurse picked up the phone. Once I identified myself, she said that Rob had passed peacefully the day before. He died at his easel while working on a landscape that was to have been a gift to his pastor. I was speechless, tears silently flowing down my face. I did not share anything with anyone for a while, but went back to my office and sat in front of the painting, still crying. I did not have the courage to call Yvonne. Later I learned details of the service from the nurse, told my resident, and we decided to attend together.

When I got home that evening, I shared the news with Nik, who was quiet as we hugged. We spoke of the good time we had at Rob's home. I shared how I used the painting for orientation. We spoke about treasuring the time we had and the gifts we received, the books, the paintings, and most importantly, the friendship.

The service was beautiful, a celebration of a wonderful human being indeed. When the bagpipes played I could not fight back the tears any longer. I said not a word to Yvonne, but we held each other in a tight embrace to convey our emotions.

## Lasting Impressions

I am grateful that my son had the privilege of sharing a game of chess with the great player. That brief encounter with Rob and his wife made a lasting impression on Nik and touched his life in a significant way. It was the first of Nik's experiences of witnessing suffering. Before then, he had never been around people who were unwell. After that encounter, Nik and Natasha both volunteered at the Program of All-Inclusive Care for the Elderly (PACE). Patients were picked up in the morning, driven to the PACE center, then returned to their homes in the evening. My son also became friends with a young boy who had cerebral palsy.

Becoming acquainted with Rob that day, and having a mutually meaningful conversation, evoked in Nik a feeling of care for others—a spark that today is a steady, burning fire on the hearth of my son's heart. His experience with Rob became the impetus for him to pursue health care. I heard from Yvonne that when Nik entered medical school, he wrote her a letter of thanks for that memorable day.

Nik's ability to listen to and connect with his family, friends, colleagues, and patients grew during medical school. I heard the compassion and care in his voice when he shared his clinical experiences on our near-daily phone calls as he walked back home. I treasure these conversations and am proud and comforted by how he values the human being and not just the disease plaguing the human body. Nik continues to give back with a listening ear, a warm hug, and even academically in a unique way. Making clear notes of his study methods and organization plans in medical school, he would make copies and share them freely to any who asked. These notes became widely known as "Pandouts" and are fondly remembered by his classmates. More recently, as a surgical senior resident, he wrote an op-ed for first-year residents titled "Dear Intern."[1]

HOUSE CALLS ARE MORE common in the realms of palliative care and hospice, but not in everyday medicine. The house calls with Rob and Yvonne were something I did on an impulse. Inviting residents and my children to share in such moments was a way to show that we don't have to segregate our hearts from our work. While this was the first house call I made in America, it most certainly wasn't my last.

*Don't be so afraid to color outside the lines that you never pick up your crayon.*

UNKNOWN

## 9  WALKING IN A PATIENT'S SHOES

*If you can learn a simple trick, Scout, you'll get along a lot
better with all kinds of folks. You never really understand
a person until you consider things from his point of view,
until you climb inside of his skin and walk around in it.*

ATTICUS FINCH IN *TO KILL A MOCKINGBIRD*

I MET a patient in the early 2000s I called Miss Connie who
was coming to the clinic for management of her hypertension.
Connie was an amazing woman, very articulate. Her accent was
immaculate. She taught English as a second language for
undergrads at the University of Tennessee. She brought apples
and candied walnuts or cashews into the clinic for Christmas.
Connie was well read, and I'd often ask what she was reading.
Despite rheumatoid arthritis that had deformed her hands, she
did calligraphy and still crocheted. When the resident who
treated her regularly was graduating, Connie crocheted the
most beautiful scarf for his wife. Connie had once been a news
journalist and photographer in New York City. She had moved
back to Tennessee because her parents were raised there,

although they were long deceased. She had no family, only close friends.

A few years into becoming a regular clinic patient, Connie had a mild stroke and had to walk with a cane. After another stroke she could no longer drive and had moved in with friends in a city some thirty miles away. When I saw her about four months after her second stroke, she was totally different. Never one to complain, Connie was very quiet, but not only from difficulties with her speaking and mobility.

"How are you doing, Miss Connie?" I asked her. "How do you spend your day?"

Connie told me that her friends worked and were not home during the day. This cultured woman loved going to the symphony, loved music, loved art, loved to walk. She was so remote and without public transportation.

"Miss Connie, you are depressed. You need to move back to the city." She started crying, and I too had tears.

"We'll talk to your friends. There are many assisted living places. I can help you find somewhere to live on the bus route. You can go to the museum, the library."

"Yes, I would like that!"

"I promise you I will start looking. I am going to India for two weeks, and then we'll keep working on this. Hopefully by Christmas we'll have you back in the city."

I called her before leaving for India. She was so excited.

"Dr. Panda, Dr. Panda, I'm moving into town."

A close friend of Connie's (whom I also knew) had invited Connie to live with her. I called Amie and thanked her and her husband, Steve. After my trip, I called Amie to check in. Connie had had another stroke. She was doing okay but the problem was, there were about six steps from the street to the yard and another eight or nine steps to get to the guest cottage. Amie told me she and Steve were working to address those mobility issues as a priority.

A policy in our clinic states that if a patient doesn't show up for three visits, they are dismissed with a certified letter. Each day at the end of the clinic session, we look at the list. That day my senior resident came to me at 5:30 p.m. and reviewed the names, indicating his plans for each of the "no show" patients. "And this woman needs to get the letter. She has not kept her appointment multiple times." He had just named Connie. I could feel a little frustration and anger rising in me, but I kept it quiet. I had an idea.

"What are you doing on Monday?" I asked him.

"I'm on the clinic rotation," he replied.

"I need you to come with me at four o'clock Monday afternoon. We're going somewhere."

## Bringing Back the Black Bag

I took him to meet Miss Connie. We climbed the very steep steps to get to the guest cottage. As a physician preceptor for residents, I evaluate my residents in all six ACGME competencies, such as professionalism, communication, knowledge, and so on. [1] The look on his face was enough to see that he realized why Miss Connie had not come to the clinic.

That's when I said to myself, I'm going to get every resident to do house calls. To see a patient in their environment is priceless. That's when I started the Bringing Back the Black Bag project with a co-faculty in the department. She too had prior experience and a passion for the importance of holistic patient care. Our home health facility leader was kind enough to give us an experienced nurse and transportation for assistance. The residents, going in pairs, had to complete at least four to six house calls in a year. I identified patients in zip codes within a ten-mile radius of the hospital who were above sixty-five years old or who had mobility issues for any reason. And it was literally a black bag we carried.

We studied the education impact on the residents and the perceptions of the patients receiving the house calls. We also published and presented the information both regionally and nationally. During our research a patient interviewed about the Black Bag project told us, "It's better than sliced bread."

The project rippled out beyond house calls. My senior resident and Miss Connie developed a friendship, so much so that he was inspired to help her feel productive. We put our heads together and got a contract with the YMCA. Twice a month in the afternoon we'd drive her and some residents to the neighborhood elementary school and we all read to the little children. Afterwards, we'd often stop at Starbucks. Once I asked her, "What would you like to have today? How about a white chocolate mocha?"

She was quick to correct me. "Dr. Panda, white chocolate is not chocolate."

One year, Natasha and I took Miss Connie shopping at Christmas. It was truly an eye opener for me. How do you buy clothes for a lady who can't zip up and button clothes? I was so proud of my daughter for her gentle yet respectful way of navigating Connie as though she had known her for a long time. They joked and laughed and shared their love for movies, especially Sex in the City. I expressed my surprise, "Miss Connie, you watch that too? Now I feel I need to see what this is all about!" The two responded instantly as one voice, "No, it is not for you!" I never did watch the series, but Natasha had Miss Connie watching her favorite Bollywood movies after that. (Natasha has a unique perception about people. Her ability to relate to children is also amazing. They love her because she can talk to them at their level; she calms them. She was a favorite at the children's museum and rehab center where she volunteered during her school holidays.)

After almost three years, we could no longer do the Black Bag program. Such visits were too time-consuming. A regular house visit was very detailed, addressing many holistic aspects of their life. In addition to a detailed physical exam, with the patient's permission we reviewed the food in their refrigerator, checked their medicine cabinet, made sure their home was safe from rugs to trip over or noted if a ramp was needed or grab-bars in the bathroom. Residents could only commit to seeing two patients instead of six during a usual clinic afternoon. The nurse could no longer be committed to us as a resource. And the commitment dwindled. It was hard to sustain financially. My co-faculty had to cut back hours and I couldn't do it alone. I would have to look for another way for residents to have that experience.

I continued to see Miss Connie until she went on hospice, even though the house calls program had long since ended. She died in 2017. Amie listed me as family in Connie's obituary.

I couldn't attend Connie's funeral because of a speaking commitment. Amie said, "Connie would be upset if you changed your plans to be at her funeral." I knew that was true. I wrote up what I wanted to say and someone else read it at the funeral. A few weeks later, Amie gave me a framed quote that Connie had created in calligraphy. She said, "Connie would like you to have this." It sits by my computer where I look at it often: *That which we love we come to resemble.*

## Making Tough Choices

So much of medical school and residency is focused on iden-tifying disease and prescribing a course of action to address the diagnosis. But what happens when the "right" answer doesn't mesh with the real world? Working at a Level 1 hospi-tal, the only safety net hospital in the region, most of the patients I care for are plagued with the social determinants of health, including poverty, lack of health insurance, low education, drug and alcohol abuse, unresolved childhood or recent trauma, domestic violence, gun violence, just to name a few.

Consider a patient admitted to the hospital for complications from uncontrolled diabetes mellitus. It is common for her to receive the following instructions at discharge: a prescription of various appropriate medications, plus instructions to eat nutritious foods and get thirty minutes of exercise daily. Those instructions feel impossible to a person living on food stamps, who has no transportation and is caring for two children while trying to keep a job in a grocery store, paying house rent, and living in a zip code where it's not even safe to go outside of the house!

It is difficult for most medical students and many physicians to relate to the environment of their patients, and that lack of understanding makes it hard for them to provide patient-centered care. *How can we best articulate to our learners that the patient population we care for really needs a lot more than a prescription or undergoing a procedure?*

This was the driving question behind the launch of a unique interactive simulation program that I started with the help of a committed interprofessional team of diverse health care professionals. We called it Walking in a Patient's Shoes. It flips the script by having young medical professionals try to follow 'the doctor's orders' while navigating a host of issues ranging from a lack of transportation and funds to unsafe environments and food deserts.

Many medical students and residents had never personally experienced the types of tough choices faced by a lot of patients seen in clinical practice. Putting learners in their patients' shoes drives home the impact that social determinants play on compliance with follow-up care. Lived experience works in a way that didactic lectures hadn't been able to achieve previously—and that we could no longer provide in person the way we had during the Bringing Back the Black Bag program.

The interactive learning experience also helps meet a number of quality and accreditation goals for both the university and hospital, including fostering holistic, patient-centered care; providing future physicians with enhanced knowledge and tools to improve population health; and addressing key hospital metrics such as readmissions and length of stay, which are significantly impacted by adherence to a medical plan.

Residents and students are given the exact clinical scenario of a patient presented upon admission and the actual discharge instructions provided to that patient and the patient's budget. Other useful details are found in the patient's social history, with all identifying details removed to ensure patient privacy. They are told the patient's social history around work, transportation needs, family support, and biweekly wages. Based on this information, the learners must navigate the four weeks of time between a patient's discharge and the scheduled follow-up appointment.

We typically schedule about two hours for this simulation. Different stations are set up to mimic the grocery store, the bank, pharmacy, physical therapy, transportation office, clinic, and so on. The students and residents work in teams, and for the simulation, each week is equal to fifteen minutes. The team has one hour to "walk in a patient's shoes" for four weeks. The second hour is for reflection and the debrief.

As a team they review the discharge instructions and strategize a plan of living. They have to review the daily requirements of living, such as grocery shopping, rent payment, child care, pharmacy bill, and so on. We intentionally give surprise scenarios, such as a sick child who cannot be left at daycare or their car breaks down, meaning that unless alternate arrangements are made, a day at work is lost.

"Do you pay the rent, or do you pay a babysitter so you can go to work? Do you choose not take your insulin this month because the car unexpectedly broke down and your income needs to go toward repairs?" These are questions that require making difficult choices.

## Walking Your Talk

After the conclusion of this interactive first hour, we give prompts for individual and group reflections. While debriefing the experience, students have an opportunity for shared learnings, education about community resources that might be available to help patients address barriers, and rethinking how we could lay out a treatment plan that more realistically mirrored a patient's specific circumstances.

Student reactions are varied to the Walking in a Patient's Shoes experience. While most learners find the session valuable and are engaged in a stimulating discussion, others keep quiet or appear disinterested. My goal is not to change or convert anyone, only to provide as best we can a glimpse into a fragment of our patients' reality.

As health care professionals, we often feel profound powerlessness against an imposing and immovable system. We have constant feelings of "I cannot do anything—the upstream forces are too powerful." This feeling is multiplied when we care for patients impacted adversely by the lack of access or other social determinants of health. The interactive Walking In a Patient's Shoes experience creates a feeling of community, so that instead of feeling powerless, our response becomes "What can we do together?"

One answer: We can organize toward collective action. Writing in the *New England Journal of Medicine*, Leo Eisenstein, then a fourth-year medical student, cites a connection between physician burnout and the experience of caring for marginalized patients.[2] One remedy is to get involved in change-making, but should political advocacy be a professional obligation for physicians, on top of everything else we are tasked with doing?

He writes, "Beyond whether we must or should do it for our patients, collective advocacy to address the harmful social determinants of health can buoy physicians' morale and thus be an act of self-care; organizing toward collective action means looking after both our patients and ourselves."

Bringing Back the Black Bag project and taking my residents on house calls was an immediate, visceral way of developing empathy for patients. Walking in a Patient's Shoes at least gave my learners new insights with a two-hour simulation. All that time I was functioning as an educator. But then I had an even more personal experience of empathy, not as a physician walking in a patient's shoes, but in my own shoes as a patient's mother.

---

*It is the capacity to feel consuming grief and pain and despair that also allows me to embrace love and joy and beauty with my whole heart. I must let it all in.*

ANNA WHITE

## 10 FACE TO FACE

*I think we all have empathy. We may not have enough
courage to display it.*

MAYA ANGELOU

IN THE DRESSING room of a department store, my daughter
was trying on dresses for her upcoming high school prom.
Suddenly, Natasha stopped in front of the mirror, eyes wide.
"Mom, what's this?" In an instant, our pleasant moment we had
anticipated for years became an occasion for panic. Distress-
ingly obvious to me was a lime-size bulge under the skin of her
left breast.

I tried not to appear overly concerned and kept a calm
demeanor. I forced myself not to think of the "C" word, and
above all, not to panic in front of my daughter. "Sit down. Let
me feel it." Not to be too obvious with my traditional and
approved method of palpating the breast, I was thorough,
checking the lymph nodes under her armpit and her other
breast. "Mom, the lump is right here, what are you doing?
That's ticklish!"

"Just checking. We'll keep an eye on it," I said, attempting nonchalance. "That dress looks great. Stand up so I can see what it looks like with your heels on."

Stepping out of the dressing room while she tried on a different dress, I pulled my cell phone from my pocket. I made an appointment with a breast surgeon with whom I worked closely at my institution. I respected him as a trusted, experienced, and wise physician.

## Daughters Aren't Data

In the days before the appointment, I noticed a growing anger in myself as I went over the medical literature. I watched this elegant, beautiful, fifteen-year old lady, thinking, *This could not be happening to my baby.* Mentally doing the math, I tried calculating odds ratios. I tried calculating the pretest probabilities for the worst diagnosis using evidenced-based medicine (EBM). I knew the data, but this "N of 1" was my daughter! I was scared, needing definite answers and reassurance, not probability.

My anger catalyzed me to question not only the way we physicians practice evidenced-based medicine in this country, but also the way I teach it. My anger was directed toward the practice of medicine, specifically how we communicate with patients, and in large part toward myself—I too was guilty.

When I completed medical school in India in the early 1980s, a specific EBM curriculum was a novelty. We were taught EBM along with clinical decision-making and individualizing patient-care decisions. A decade later, when I repeated an internal medicine residency in America, it was commonplace to teach and apply evidenced-based medicine. As an educator, I know that EBM is the prime means of educating and practicing medicine scientifically to achieve safer, consistent, and cost-effective care. But where do human touch and relationships fit into evidence-based medicine? Even though application of evidence is a core skill in training future physicians, there are companion components to the holistic care of the individual patient who are entrusted to us. Understanding EBM goes beyond the single E of *evidence* as we enter into a partnership management plan with a patient. I propose that physicians must master many more E's.

## Empathy-Based Medicine Means Many E's

Empathy is integral to the patient/physician relationship. Am I aware and perceptive of my patients' emotions, or when more face-to-face time is needed, or am I scared to show my own emotional vulnerability? Do I use the need to rush to complete the next electronic task as an excuse? Empathy builds relationships and partnerships, and *empathy*-based medicine must be coupled with the existing evidenced-based practice.[1]

*Emotions* are part of being human. I know that honoring my own emotions as a physician is critical to my own self-care and is vital to building a caring relationship with my patients and colleagues. Physicians often fear appearing weak for showing emotions. Bottled up emotions come out as untoward behavior if we don't have a healthy outlet for them. I've found it is good to balance boundaries and emotions, while bravely revealing my humanness. At sad or happy moments when patients cry, it's not uncommon for my tears to come too.

A partnership starts with the *expectations* we have for ourselves and our patients, as well as what our patients and their families expect from us. Unrealistic expectations can lead to frustration for both parties. Expectations need to be openly stated and recognized for a true partnership.

I admit I had expectations as a parent and a physician. I wanted my daughter's surgeon to have treated hundreds of cases like hers, to sit down, inquire about our needs, and take time to explain every detail, consoling as needed.

Three days after prom dress shopping, I sat with my daughter in the surgeon's office. For the first time in many years, I was on a new side of the desk. "It's definitely larger than we'd expect," he said, "so I do need to do an ultrasound and take a biopsy." He did so the same day, and I remember how he was very gentle. It was hard for me to see her in pain. "We'll get the biopsy back soon," he said, professional, yet also kind and open. He talked to me as a patient's mother—not as another physician.

And I asked questions like a mother and not as his colleague. "What do you think? What is your experience with this type of condition?" I honed in on his facial expressions, his eyes, and his body language. Was he smiling, grim, thinking of something else? The one person in front of us was my child. All my senses were on high alert. I was focused as I had never been before, adrenaline pumping, and my world was nothing except these few moments.

My daughter and I had our own emotions and concerns: *Can I go to my prom? What does this mean for my life? Will she need cosmetic surgery? Do I need to re-think her going off to college?* The surgeon gave me space to ask questions without feeling foolish. He listened, unhurried.


THE *ETHICS*, cultural upbringing, and beliefs of patients and their family also influence how much they hear or want to hear. In America, patient autonomy is the cornerstone of medical ethics. I remember my days in India when often families would demand, "Please don't tell mother the diagnosis, she will die; don't take away her hope." I wanted the surgeon to understand my ethics and frame his manner in context of my cultural values.

*Engagement* and *empowerment* of the patient and family are critical. Is the family partnered with the patient in their care? Is the patient engaged in their own care? Have we taken the necessary time with them to facilitate engagement, or do we act as if we have all the answers? The physician must initiate this partnership, empowering them where they can feel safe and bravely share vulnerabilities. They tell their life story allowing us to offer what they need for healing.

I often wonder, how do we measure the *effort* of care providers? Time spent during intake and long hours spent off the clock researching a patient's background can yield pertinent answers not printed on an EBM report. Thus, applying EBM may prove premature.

Physicians must also initiate the team effort; no one can do it alone. Our surgeon ensured that his nurse was accessible to us. She was knowledgeable, had a teen daughter, and had time to communicate with us.


*EDUCATION, experience* and *empirical* observations of physicians in their diagnosis process are also invaluable E's. Not every patient follows a study or a textbook. I wanted my daughter's surgeon to have seen hundreds of similar cases in girls her age.

Recognizing my capacity for *error* as a physician must be taken into consideration with every diagnosis. Physicians are human, and our past mistakes often determine how we interpret evidence. I have made errors, and they have been my most powerful teachers. I can never forget the time I failed to stop an antibiotic on a patient. Saving the patient impaired his hearing, but I should have stopped it sooner. Now I am hypervigilant about side effects of medications.

We must also consider *equity*, which includes the patient's *environmental* influences prior to applying evidence. I often see patients admitted to the hospital in advanced stages of illness, long overdue for effective treatment. Was that because early access to health care was not easily available? Other patients arrive in the emergency room having recently lived in areas of the world lacking access to clean water, healthy foods, or basic hygiene.

Equity also includes a patient's *economic* situation, a point which cannot be underestimated. Even though we may have access to several excellent action plans, the health care system may not allow us to proceed, or the patient may have insufficient resources to pay for treatment. We must accept feasibility considering patient affordability and ease. I work in a not-for-profit critical access hospital where we are tied by the resources available. I have to choose medications based on what patients can afford.

I don't want to negate the importance of *evidence*. But evidence is not valuable until you consider the whole patient in front of you. Evidence has its maximum impact when applied in the context of these other E's: empathy, emotions, expectations, ethics, engagement, empowerment, effort, education, experience, error, equity, environment, economics. And when sufficient evidence isn't available, how can expert opinion provide a viable way forward?

## A Team Approach to Empathy

My main point is to lay groundwork that guides us to ask this important question: Are we providing thorough, thoughtful, well-rounded training for our future physicians? We start teaching medical students on day-one of their training how to take a medical history; it's something they'll do the rest of their career. Let's train them to ask about those other E's. *Where do you get your medications? What do you do for a living? Where do you get your social support?* Learning EBM (with all the E's), is like any other new skill clinicians must learn—by practice, by iteration, by accepting that juggling all the E's is impossible to do perfectly. There's no right way to do it. Each clinician should develop their own style.

Am I, as an educator and clinician, making certain that I and the learners on my team address more of these E's before definitively applying the evidence? In the current health care environment of time poverty, this responsibility should not overburden us. We can engage our team members to take ownership for pursuing different E's. Let us as a team educate our learners about the other professionals available to provide patient-centered-care.

Physicians and health care providers are committed to life-long learning, accepting that continuous education is a must. At different stages of training, we may find it easier and more appropriate to practice the various E's in our roles. Medical students closest to the patient have more time and are not called upon for other skills compared to their interns. They may be better able to understand their patient's story with empathy. The senior resident preparing for boards is the steward of evidence. The senior attending can offer experience and expert opinion. I feel grateful for the clinician-scientists who find new ways to engage, enable, and empower shared-care. Case managers maybe best at advocating economic- and environment-based practices, having knowledge regarding resource needs. Physical therapists constantly consider patient environments. In Natasha's case, our surgeon ensured team care. His nurse was especially accessible and knowledgeable.

It takes an interprofessional team to provide true patient-centered care. Physicians are the conductors of this orchestra for harmonious patient care. We must know when and who to ask for help as we incorporate all these E's into the rituals we teach and practice.

Each patient—and every physician—has a body and a soul living together in sickness and in health. I venture the thought that sometimes the way we treat patients separates body from soul. Empathy-based medicine, in light of the other E's, is the model that provides a way for us to take care of all the needs of our patients.

MY DAUGHTER'S breast cancer scare was in 2006. The lump was benign. In 2008 she found a second lump, also benign. By God's infinite grace, today Natasha is healthy and well. My own journey through those times as her mother paved how I practice and teach empathy-based *and* evidence-based medicine.

⌒

*Empathy is not simply a matter of trying to imagine what others are going through, but having the will to muster enough courage to do something about it. In a way, empathy is predicated upon hope.*

CORNEL WEST

# PART 3

# HOW DO I HEAL AS I STRIVE TO SERVE?

*You can survive on your own; you can grow strong on your own; you can prevail on your own; but you cannot become human on your own.*

FREDERICK BUECHNER

## 11 FAMILY DOESN'T MEAN BLOOD

*It's like everyone tells a story about themselves inside their own head. Always. All the time. That story makes you what you are. We build ourselves out of that story.*

PATRICK ROTHFUSS

DIFFICULTIES CAN OFTEN SERVE as doors that invite us to come inside and to look within ourselves. We have the choice of opening the door, stepping over the threshold, and learning what is offered there; cracking the door a bit and immediately shutting it again in favor of the status quo; or wrenching the door wide and flinging it back on its hinges in a fearful reaction of anger or defiance. I had the incredible blessing of walking inside one such door during an overpoweringly troublesome time.

In 2007 I found myself in a dark and lonely place. I was facing a significant personal loss, divorce, that came abruptly, leaving a void and a desperate plea for the earth to envelop me. The details are private, as Terry Tempest Williams once wrote, "not as a secret but as a prayer." I don't know any human being who goes through life without facing an event that brings them to their knees, whether that is depression, death, divorce, disease, or another form of despair over the unexpected heart-wrenching moments of life.

I would get up, go to work. I would function as a professional who is trained to compartmentalize her own life's challenges. I would then come home and crawl into bed, often skipping dinner. I lost a lot of weight.

It was precisely the Multiple Hats Syndrome! I simply did not want to think about anything personal. To do so was distracting and painful. But if I had been more open, authentic, and had asked for help, perhaps I could have integrated my learnings sooner. Perhaps it would have been an easier, less bumpy journey. I wouldn't have been so lonely. Our inner and outer lives cannot be compartmentalized—they are really one and the same.

## Don't Worry, I Will Always Hold Your Hand

Natasha returned to Chattanooga from Boston University to take care of me. Nik had just begun college at the University of Virginia. In my suffering, I transferred much of my frustration and anger onto Natasha. Sometimes she took it silently, but at other times she was firm about her message of support for me. For instance, one day she turned *The Kardashians* on TV, and I lashed out, "I do not want to watch this! It's such a waste of time." She fired right back, "Mom, you just have to see that there are crazy things in the world. You can't always be serious!" Another day she said, "Mom, just get out of bed. Stop having a pity party."

As Natasha and I were talking one day, I expressed my lingering loneliness. My daughter emphatically but caringly said, "Mom, family doesn't mean blood! You just need to get over this and learn to be your own best friend." I listened to this wisdom from my child. From that point on, I saw things differently and was able to refocus my priorities.

Family doesn't mean blood. This revelation at such a low juncture in my life reminded me of another time when my daughter, as a young child, demonstrated her considerable strength and protective character. We were living in Yonkers. Our bedtime routine included me lying down between my son and daughter as we read stories and said our prayers. On one of these nights, rain crashed about, heavy and wild. My little son was afraid, and I said to Nik, "How about this—why don't you hold my hand." Natasha spoke out clearly in the dark, "Mommy, don't worry, I will always hold your hand. Don't be scared."

Family doesn't mean blood. Natasha's words became a mantra that prompted me to see who fortified me through my soul's dark night. Let me tell you about these people I call my angels.

## You Can and You Will

At times of loss and confusion, no matter our age, it seems our inner child needs someone to reach out with reassurance. For me, that someone was a beloved teacher who showed me how to find my inner resources more than once—as a child and again in 2007.

When I was a young girl in fourth grade, I felt I could always go and talk to my teacher, Miss Judy, and she would know the answer. She listened even to the most trivial childhood matters with her beautiful eyes, her young yet knowing heart, and her finely tuned ears.

I was struggling with peer pressure and jealousy, not being accepted by the elite group of girls in my school. The girls would huddle, talk and laugh. I felt intimidated. They were slim and pretty; I wanted to be like them. Those were the same years I was reading Archie comics, and I was fascinated with Betty and Veronica. I wanted to be Veronica. She was so popular. I was heartbroken that I couldn't fit in with the elite clique at school. They would intentionally invite other girls to join their group, but I never got an invitation.

I would ask my mom to make food they liked and take it to them. I wanted to win them over. One day, they had a picnic and I wasn't invited. I went to Miss Judy in tears. "I do everything I can think of to be part of their group, but I don't know why they don't like me." She said, "Mukta, you are too open. Sometimes you don't have to share everything."

Another time I went to Miss Judy in tears complaining over a disagreement with a classmate. Without a word, she took pencil to paper, and then handed it to me. I read a mystery: *I complained I had no shoes until I saw a man with no feet.*

The words themselves held little meaning to my young mind, but I trusted my teacher enough for the paper to hold a place of honor taped to my bedroom mirror. This succinct Persian proverb was the first lesson in what would become a life-long practice of paying close attention to the wisdom of others. When the mirror could hold no more scraps of paper, I simply wrote quotes on my bedroom wall. (Fortunately, my parents did not scream at me.) As I matured, I gradually peeled back the layers of the fruit my beloved teacher offered me that day: *Be intentionally thankful for all your blessings.*

This one simple but profound lesson has stayed with me all through the years as it continues to reveal even more levels of meaning that inform my life. I love sharing quotes with people. I even wrote a book with my dad in 2017 titled *Rhythm of Our Hearts* that is a compilation of quotes and our reflections, based on a group email series I started after my kids left for college.

Shoes have also become a symbol of blessing and a source of joy. I am mindful of the shoes on my feet each day as I walk through this journey of life, asking questions and paying attention to answers. Because I wear my physician's white coat, I use funky-colored shoes to make a statement. (Mary Janes and oxfords with ties are my go-to shoes.) I never knew what shoes to wear to prepare myself for this journey, but through different experiences in life, I have said, "Wear the shoes that make you happy and the terrain will teach you how to tread on the journey—even if it is unknown to you."

A remarkable teacher, Miss Judy gave me the sense of confidence to stand in the world with courage in spite of differences. I learned how to be in a team of young people from widely varying cultures, traditions, religions, languages, and interests. She taught us how to listen to others' stories and to reflect upon them. I always felt more appreciated and better about myself in her presence and I suspect my classmates did, too. She taught us about purposeful service. We celebrated our successes and also our failures, and we learned from our mistakes. She embraced us and accepted us all. I try to emulate these learnings, especially in my relationships.

I am still friends with my fourth-grade teacher, Miss Judy. To this day, we enjoy being together with every trip I make to India. When I was in great inner turmoil in my personal life in 2007, she was there for me. She understood what I had been going through.

When I gathered the courage to share the loss with Miss Judy, she said, "Mukta, this has torn your heart. This is worse than death. You must have faith and you will get through. You can and you will."

*You can and you will.* Miss Judy had given me more words to live by.


## Soul Sisters

When I was about twelve, a new girl close to my age climbed aboard the bus on the way to school. What I noticed at first glance was not her straight black hair, large, expressive eyes, or smiling face, but her shoes. Oxford lace-ups were not exactly a tradition in my part of the world, but this girl wore them, complete with the prerequisite white socks that would later become familiar footwear in England. Our eyes met and there was an immediate connection. It was as if the two of us became soul sisters in that moment.

Three short years following the day we met on the bus, Indrani moved away. As a result of her father's military service, she was already widely traveled and well-spoken. From afar, she would write faithfully, page after page. She even penned an entire travel journal as a gift for me. I wrote back perhaps three lines, but I still have her beautiful journal. She created poetry and all sorts of extemporaneous pieces. This voracious reader, who shared freely her poems, photos, and current reading list, helped me by way of lively discussion to understand the world of literature in a fuller light.

I admired and envied my friend's creative gifts, but thankfully was able to turn my envy into an asset after discovering how easily we complemented each other. Whereas I lacked a background in classical literature and its applications for life, she had not spent concentrated time with mathematics and science. I gravitated toward the scientific intricacies of the natural world; her inclinations were literary and artistic. Thus, our interests and abilities dove-tailed each other in close bonds of mutual respect.

Indrani and I were pen pals for decades, until finally we met again in 2006. My family had gone to London to celebrate New Year's Eve and so we took a trip to Sweden to visit Indrani. Ever since, we travel together every year to places like England, Italy, Japan, Hungary, India. She plans our trips. I just show up. She makes beautiful scrapbooks afterwards.

I have this amazing person who shares life through prose, quotes, literature, and pictures. I reap the benefits. Still today, every morning she sends me one of her photographs. As I was first writing this chapter, she even sent me a photo of a splash of water she'd spilled on her floor and it looked like the silhouette of an angel. It felt like playful confirmation that the angels who befriend us during our lives are truly divine gifts.

Family doesn't mean blood. Belonging doesn't always require presence in person. Community comes from the connections we develop across time and place. Friendship sustains me and helps me heal through the hardest of times, and in happy times, too.

## Aunty and Uncle

When my father was in the Middle East for an extended time, my mother continued her internist work at home in Goa. One of the patients in Mummy's department had been hospitalized for a prolonged time and remained in critical condition. Mummy was in communication with his young wife, Sunanda. It was after her husband succumbed to his illness that Sunanda expressed the desire for work within our home. She needed income so that her three children could have an education. Mummy's solution was to help her with a home and the means to educate the children. We called her Aunty and she stayed with us in our home.

Aunty was hard-working and determined indeed. She took care of our home and we always looked forward to coming home to a delicious meal cooked with love. We were always greeted with a smile and care. She wanted to know about our day. Her interest felt warm and genuine, and it was easy to speak with her. After I left India, I missed her. Before I moved to the United States, I went to India with my young children for a long visit. I knew it would be a few years before I could visit home again. Aunty took us under her wing, pampering us by cooking the wonderful dishes we loved and making sure I had plenty of rest.

That was thirty years ago. After my brothers and I left home, Sunanda Aunty educated herself and was employed in a respectable job at the same hospital where she lost her husband and first met my parents. She retired in 2018. Sunanda Aunty is now a proud grandmother of five grandchildren. Her own children are educated and well settled. I communicate with her via phone and her daughter, Tilotma, via the modern WhatsApp. Whenever I visit home in Goa, she is sure to have all my favorite dishes ready. Her whole family greets us with love and care.

MY FATHER CLAIMS he has three brothers, two being biological and one destined, Keshkamat Uncle, as I call him. His family is our family. Uncle worked at the bank in Panjim, Goa, where my dad went to open an account soon after arriving in Goa in August 1969. Uncle must have sensed Papa was new, coming up to him and asking Papa if he needed help. That spontaneous act of kindness sparked a friendship that has grown and blessed us in every part of our lives, not just my parents and all our family, but especially me and my children.

I know Uncle is just a phone call or a WhatsApp message away. He continues to be a silent force of strength, reliance, and trust and an intercessor in prayer for us. We are reassured that while Uncle is there in Goa, we have nothing to worry about.

My Aunty and Uncle are people I have always been able to rely on, even sometimes more than my own family. These two individuals and their generous care remind me that family is not blood.

## Angels in the Office

By walking through that dark time with love from my grown children, my parents, and my lifelong trusted friends, I became braver in reaching out to my colleagues in a more intimate way. Because I was feeling so lost and vulnerable—yet supported—I found a deeper appreciation for and openness to friendship.

I was able to see how some of my colleagues had been *sent* to me as messengers of God's care. Up until then, I had seen them as friends from my department. We had close, pleasant working relationships and would enjoy chats about our families, faith, and our activities. It was a comfortable arrangement, but God knew I needed more.

Some of the young professionals who were present for me were former students; others were residents, colleagues, and soul sisters. They perceived that something was wrong, but never probed. Small gifts began quietly appearing on my desk throughout the day—a piece of chocolate, an encouraging note or quote—touches of kindness that surprised me and lifted my spirits. One day a piece of pottery came with the inscription, "If He hands it to you, He will handle it for you." Further along, a colleague's mother gave me a devotional book called *Streams in the Desert,* which has become so influential that I still read from it daily.

Sometimes, colleagues moved away for further training and returned as faculty. I had a special connection with one person in particular about my daughter's age. She is an interesting blend of worldly naivety coupled with spiritual maturity, and I enjoy our philosophical conversations even today. Her care for my whole family, especially my parents, is genuine and visible in every gesture, whether small or large.

The lenses through which I viewed my friends were changing, refining, and gaining a sharper focus. These compassionate teammates walked that journey with me. We had always prayed for each other, but now we developed a soul connection as we held each other's hands and prayed in a more meaningful way. One colleague in particular continues to be my "walking partner" on a journey of spiritual, emotional, and physical healing.

While my children were there to support me, they too needed support. These messengers were also there for my children. Each time one of us would falter or need encouragement, the right person arrived to provide. One of the four individuals who had been sent to stand and walk beside me became close friends with my daughter. Every one of us felt loved and cared for by these angels who surrounded and reached out to us as extensions of God's hands.

HOW GRATEFUL I am to those who showed me how to live out of faith and trust and who provided me with a mirror of compassionate community. By sharing their own journey, these angels became my role models in surrender. Conceptually I understood the idea of unconditional surrender, but hadn't actually practiced it. Seeing the personal experience of this quality of unconditional surrender in others gave me the chance to live what I knew.

———

*God's angel sets up a circle of protection around us while*
    *we pray.*

PSALM 34:7

# 12 TURNING POINTS

*You cannot change your destination overnight, but you can change your direction overnight.*

JIM ROHN

IN 2007 I was questioning my purpose, value, and worth, and wondering where I belonged. I was also struggling professionally. The politics and expectations that came with the role as a physician leader in education often seemed misaligned with my values and gifts. When I had first taken on the role nine years earlier, it was with the goals of nurturing young physicians and growing the faculty team, both in size and in their sense of collaboration. Over time, I felt the role had come to demand more focus on fiscal issues, less on relationship. And that's not who I am.

It was a rough period both at home and at work. I could hardly open my mouth without crying. I didn't want to speak with anybody. And yet I had to put up a brave front.

I was so distressed that I had written a resignation letter. My parents have never told me directly what to do, but have instead always asked open, honest questions so that I may interpret my answers for myself and make my own choices. That was the only time my dad gave me advice, "Don't submit your resignation. Don't give up something that you already have." He also added, "When a sand storm comes, what do the palm trees do? They remain still and bow their heads. We need to be still and avoid the sand going into our eyes and mouth." Because my dad never said something to me like this before, I respected him and honored his advice. I didn't submit my resignation.

A week after the conversations with my parents and my restless inner dialogue, I was sitting in my office staring at my computer screen when the phone rang. My assistant informed me that I had a call from the Accreditation Council of Graduate Medical Education (ACGME). I jolted upright because this was very unusual, not common, and never had I heard of or faced being called personally by the ACGME. It could only mean one of two things, either good news or not good news!

As I picked up the phone I heard, "Congratulations!" The voice identified himself as David Leach, who was then CEO and president of the ACGME. He was calling to tell me that I was a recipient of the Parker J. Palmer Courage to Teach award. The award recognizes medical educators for their dedication to teaching physicians and their talent for creating innovative and effective residency programs. I stared in silence and disbelief.

I had just collapsed from my personal loss, so receiving the honor felt almost incongruent. *Now I'm getting this award? What does this mean?*

After a few minutes I called my parents. It must have been about 2:00 a.m. in India. I do not remember the conversation, but I know there were tears, lots of them. That night, I was copied on an email to my dean in the department of medicine, and I soon received an email with his congratulations.

## Retreat and Reflect

One of the benefits of the Parker J. Palmer Courage to Teach award was the opportunity to attend a retreat. I knew a physician at another institution who received the award in a previous year. I called to ask him about it and he said, "Congratulations! Don't miss the retreat. That is the best part of this award."

Looking forward to the weekend retreat on my calendar gave me hope. Then the retreat itself was a pivotal moment.

I arrived at the Fetzer Institute where the retreat was held, unsure of what to expect. The emails beforehand from our facilitators were warm, simply inviting attendees to take a short interlude from our demanding work and spend it in retreat with our co-awardees. I did not know any of the awardees. I had a room to myself, overlooking a garden. There was no TV, no internet access, but a journal and a flashlight on the table. The surroundings had a calming effect.

As we met the first evening for dinner and the beginning of our time together, the setting was not something I had seen since I left India. We had seats of different types, some straight back, others cushioned, and some low cushions on the floor arranged in a circle. A low table with a candle in the center completed the serene atmosphere. My time at the retreat is difficult to describe in words. It was an experience I felt with all my senses. It was an experience that left me yearning for more.

I experienced how reflective practices with the support of community could draw forth one's insights. It was surprising and energizing to remind myself of what I had written about in my medical school application, the reasons I wanted to be in a health profession, to be a physician. I reconnected with who I saw myself as.

Our first invitation was to reflect on our inner landmarks, the kinds of experiences that represented significant moments in which our identity and integrity were encouraged, tested, or established. The invitation was not limited to the positive, productive events of our lives. Our handout specifically named times of pain and uncertainty. We could choose five or six events that felt most significant and take time to think about them. Chronology or connecting the dots was not required. The invitation was to journal, create, draw, whatever we were called to do. The invitation was liberating. I sat on the patio outside the room and stared into space. Then I drew: stick figures for my family and my friends, a map for my travels, tears for the dark time, all in a circle. As I stared at the circle, I added a lamp with a flame in the center and the rays of sun around it. Connecting lines to each of the landmarks around the circle, that was the first time I actually named that my thread was my faith!

This was the beginning. The rest of our time together was just as beautiful. I was introduced to poetry, art, and excerpts as ways to invite and assist with deep and difficult conversations. There was safety and a feeling of connection. Before the retreat, I did not have the required language or skills and did not know the art of how to have those deep and difficult conversations with myself.

## Relaxing, Rejuvenating, Rejoicing in Residency

After attending the retreat, I began holding weekly reflective sessions (or "circles of trust") with two colleagues and soon also a resident who I knew was struggling. Because I was willing to lean on my closest colleagues more, gaining strength from those relationships then gave me confidence to offer support on a broader level. It wasn't long before we made the same reflective sessions available to residents. Medical students and residents typically enter their training with intense altruism and a commitment to care for their patients. But during training, they rarely have an opportunity to reflect on their emotional experiences. We felt that lack of inner awareness might be an important cause of burnout.

To address this lack, I created a program called Relaxing, Rejuvenating, Rejoicing in Residency sessions (RRRnR). For an hour each Thursday, we would gather, without an agenda, and sit in a circle. A few moments of silence allow us to become fully present and to leave the rest of our lives behind. I would tell them, "If you have things to do, write them on a paper and tear it up. Now be present here in this room for the next thirty minutes of your life."

People would bring a book chapter, a video—anything they want to share. The session was a safe space for residents to talk about the emotional experience of being a physician. We studied the coping skills of residents who had gone through the RRRnR sessions over eighteen months. The research project was conducted with the professor of Industrial-Organizational and Occupational Health Psychology. Results showed that residents who attended at least three sessions per quarter had positive coping skills and reported lower levels of stress.[1]

Then word got around, so invitations were extended and more people came. Nurses started coming, patients and family, a pastor, a book author, the CEO, the Dean. In later years, pharmacy students and others from all different divisions within the hospital came to the sessions. I once led a very tense meeting as chair of the department and after the meeting, a colleague said, "Wow, Mukta, can we have an RRRnR session now?"

Within these RRRnR sessions, we heard each other's frustrations and discovered we could relate to each other with more empathy. This sense of community led to further collaborations and more camaraderie in our shared work. Coworkers began to feel that they had a bond, a connection with each other due to sharing in the RRRnR sessions.

My colleagues and I experienced such value thanks to these practices that eventually I went through the two-year training program to become a Circle of Trust facilitator with the Center for Courage & Renewal. I now lead various retreats, including co-facilitating the annual retreat for recipients of the ACGME Courage to Teach and Courage to Lead awards.

AT THE BACK of my mind, I always knew I was blessed, and I offered simple gratitude with my prayers. Now that I was more aware, I found I could better recognize, celebrate and truly appreciate the magnitude of my many blessings. I found a true understanding of my belief that there are no chances or coincidences, only confirmations. I now sought these, claimed them, and named them as such!

*Your ordinary acts of love and hope point to the extraordinary promise that every human life is of inestimable value.*

DESMOND TUTU

## 13  GRAY'S ANATOMY

*Wisdom is openness to wherever the path might lead and*
*empathy for the struggles and anxieties of other people*
*who are trying to figure out life, right alongside us.*

JEREMY SIERRA

BY REMAINING at the same hospital throughout my career, my life is blessed with a continuity of connection to certain patients. My first patient as a second-year resident in 1996 was a gentleman who had been transferred in critical condition from an area hospital. We knew only that he had been admitted to an outlying facility where he had presented in a state of shock after vomiting large amounts of fresh blood. The working diagnosis was severe liver damage most likely due to alcohol. Unable to stabilize him with most conventional methods at the outlying facility, he was transferred to our tertiary referral center for more advanced interventional care.

I knew the grim prognosis of a patient presenting as he had, and I lacked the experience to know any different. I also knew we had to continue with full-press treatment, enlisting all the specialists, and do that fast. Determined that I would not give up on him, I affirmed that decision in discussions with the patient's wife, who was his only immediate family member. Although we knew there was slim chance of recovery, I reassured her that although his condition necessitated end-of-life preparations, every available management option, every piece of technology and assistance at the hospital, would be employed to provide her husband the best of care.

Throughout the ensuing night, she asked me, "Doctor, what do you think?" She clearly wanted to know my realistic assessment. In turn, I never relinquished hope and continued to orchestrate everything possible in his favor.

This patient, whom I always addressed as Mr. Bryan out of respect, did improve after that tumultuous time in the critical care unit followed by a prolonged stay in the wards with intensive rehabilitation. I scheduled regular and frequent follow-up visits with me in the outpatient clinic. His wife, who insisted I call her Patricia or Pat, made sure he was compliant and came with him to every visit. I was happy with his improved medical condition. Although his disease could not be cured, it could be kept in check as long as he adhered to his medication regimen, made the necessary lifestyle changes, especially complete abstinence from alcohol.

At each visit I echoed with even sterner fervor his wife's message of absolutely no alcohol! "You were very lucky, a miracle actually," I said. "Alcohol will kill you if you restart. It is out of your system. Now we need to work on getting it out of your head." He listened and promised to comply. I explored his interests outside of being a professor and discussed options to keep himself occupied since he was now retired from teaching anatomy. He assured me he spent time with a good group of supportive friends.

## Forgiving Mistakes

At one such visit about six months after his discharge from the hospital, I realized Mr. Bryan was straining to hear me. "Speak louder," his wife said to him, then addressing me, "He seems to not hear well these days." My heart sank. I knew what it was. I was staring at his medicines and realized that I had failed to discontinue one antibiotic that was appropriately given in the acute setting but should have been stopped after a few weeks. Hearing loss was not a common but a known side effect of this medication. My face must have displayed my emotions accurately. I was frank and honest and apologized. I said that the antibiotic was the probable cause and I was unsure of how permanent the loss would be. I reassured them that I would refer him immediately to a specialist to get it checked. Both of their forgiving responses were humbling.

"No worries, doctor," he said. "I can wear a hearing aid. He proceeded to make a joking yet loving remark about how he would not have to hear his wife's nags all the time. Patricia just gave him a loving glare and shook her head chuckling. I was relieved but learned yet another valuable lesson through this E of error-based medicine. I was made acutely aware of the importance to consider every effect of each prescription in our patients' care plan.

## Fast-Forward Twelve Years

I stayed in contact with Mr. and Mrs. Bryan over the next decade or more, putting in place thorough follow-up care as needed. They were regular in their visits to the clinic. He had very occasional relapses with alcohol use and depression, but these were brief and he would recover through the support of his caring wife and his supportive community. Patricia and I would often talk separately, where she felt comfortable sharing her concerns about her husband. She had to go back to work, and they had hired a sitter to be with Mr. Bryan during the day. I think she used me as a sounding board. We often conspired together about his treatment plan before his visit to ensure we would present a united and more emphatic front.

Over the years, I found myself sharing more of my own story, talking about my family and journey to the USA. His wife spoke fondly of their niece, Angie, and her family in Chattanooga. I had met Angie and her husband during the hospitalization. Each visit they made it a point to inquire about my children and parents. If my children or I were mentioned in the local newspaper for academic or cultural achievements, then Mr. Bryan would send me a laminated copy of the paper clipping. One year when there was a tragic train accident in India, Mr. Bryan called to inquire if any of my family was affected and to offer sympathy. I always looked forward to their visits and our time together.

## Last Requests

In 2009 I was notified that Mr. Bryan had been admitted again, to the same room as before. Whenever I would stop in to see him, this thoughtful man would ask about my family by name, never failing to ask how I was doing as well. I would always ask, "Can I do anything else for you?" and only once did he make a request. He asked if I could bring him a copy of *Gray's Anatomy*, the textbook written by Henry Gray and illustrated by Henry Vandyke Carter, used widely across the globe. (Regarded as an extremely influential work on the subject, *Gray's* continues to be revised and republished from its initial publication in 1858.)

"Okay, I will get you one," I told him and soon ordered a special edition from India. I knew that this book had a special meaning for him, being an anatomy professor. We had often reminisced on how the teaching and practice of medicine had changed over the years, especially with new information burgeoning at a tremendous pace. He wondered if the *Gray's Anatomy* textbook was any different.

One day, in the middle of preparing to attend a conference in California, a message was delivered to me—Mr. Bryan had been admitted to the hospital again for a routine screening procedure. While hoping I wouldn't be late for my flight, I stopped by his room for a quick visit.

"How are you?" came his characteristic greeting.

"I am well," I responded.

"Remember *Gray's Anatomy*?"

"I am still waiting for it to arrive from India," I said, then explained about needing to catch my plane and waved good-bye.

Something slowed my steps as I rushed past the hospital's library doors. I took a deep breath and ducked in. I knew the librarian well and proceeded to her office, "Would you happen to have an extra copy of *Gray's*?" I inquired.

"Sorry," she replied, "we only keep one reference copy for the library. The rest are all digitally available."

Upon hearing our exchange from the background, a young library assistant walked up to the desk with an old copy of the prized text. Smiling, she offered it to me and revealed, "I only put it on my desk so I will look intelligent!"

You may guess how quickly I burned a path back up to my patient's room to deposit the book into his arms. As I turned to leave, Mr. Bryan beamed at me and hugged his anatomy book tightly.

I WAS on time for my flight. Attendants were giving ubiquitous instructions over the loud speaker—*turn off your devices...fasten your seat belts*. Just then my phone rang. Despite seeing that it was Patricia, I resisted picking up. I didn't turn off my phone, only set it to vibrate while I took a moment to think. I felt in my gut there must be an urgent reason. Based on our relationship and understanding for years, I knew that Patricia would not be persistent if it were not important. *Why is she not texting? Why does she keep on redialing incessantly?* These questions further fed my feelings of concern. It rang again. I knew I had to speak with her. Quickly looking around, I lowered my head, cupping my mouth, and whispered "Hello?"

"Dr. Panda, he's arrested! They are coding him! They are coding him!" The flight attendant was now in front of me, demanding I turn off the phone. I looked up at her, then looked at my phone, not sure what I was feeling or what I needed to do. I can't recall what I said when hanging up, but I can still feel the reluctance of doing so.

Much of that long, cross-country journey I spent in prayer. Upon arriving in San Francisco close to midnight, I phoned the doctor-on-call and learned that Mr. Bryan had not survived.


THE NEXT MORNING, I mustered enough courage to return Patricia's call. I said hello but then held silence. Neither of us spoke any words, but even across the miles felt each other's loss. After a long moment I said, "I am so sorry." She asked only if I would come to his memorial service. "Of course." As soon as my conference presentation was over, I cut short my stay in San Francisco. I took a red-eye flight, arriving home in the early morning on the day of the service.

My daughter happened to be in town, home from college. Both my kids knew of Mr. Bryan, as I had shared their newspaper clippings he would bring to me. I asked Natasha to come to the service with me, and she did not hesitate to say yes. I quickly showered and changed, still unsure what I would say when I saw Patricia.

## A Valuable Vessel

It was a cold crisp morning. We arrived at the church early, and I intentionally chose to sit in the back, away from the center aisle. The services flier had a smiling picture of Mr. Bryan wearing a tuxedo. I could not hold back tears as I stared at it. Then Patricia entered, standing tall, staring straight ahead to avoid eye contact. The service itself is a bit of a blur to me. Mr. Bryan was the first patient I had lost after a long relationship.

What got my attention was when the pastor talked of my patient's last moments. "I was there right before he died, and he was doing what he loved best—roaming through his *Gray's Anatomy*."

Tears streamed down my face as I sat there in the pew and thought, *What if I hadn't slowed down for that minute in front of the library? What if I hadn't responded to that inner nudge? What if I had lost that moment to be a valuable vessel?* Natasha lovingly laid her hand on my thigh.

We never know what we miss in our daily preoccupations. Only when we return to calm and stillness are we open to the workings of God's hand. I am so grateful I stopped that day to hear the small quiet voice inside that suggested I go to the library to borrow *Gray's Anatomy* for my friend.

After the service I stood in the corner, and when most everyone had left, I mustered up the courage to go and give Patricia a hug. We just held each other tight. We didn't exchange any spoken words, but our embrace spoke of our mutual loss and grief. Then I silently walked away with my daughter.

## Another Loss

Patricia remained on my mind, and I called her a few days later. It was much easier to speak across the phone lines than in person. I know that there were tears in our conversation. As we recollected the good moments and the fun times, we tried to reassure ourselves that he did not suffer at the end. And that's when I told her that she needed to start taking care of herself. I knew she had health problems of her own and was not very compliant with her own treatment regimen. I had encouraged her to find a primary care physician for herself, but was also mindful of how hard she worked both at a job and caring for her husband. Her life had centered around him. She agreed, so I later scheduled a primary care appointment for her and made sure she kept it.

We spoke regularly, and one day she asked if she could send something to me via email. It was a beautiful encouraging and inspirational paragraph. That started an email dialogue for the next few months. I would send her emails to inquire about how she was doing, often attaching a positive quote and confirming she kept her appointments. I could tell from her emails that she had started interacting more with her niece and niece's family.

I hadn't seen Patricia for several months, so we decided to have coffee and settled on a convenient day a few weeks later. A day before our scheduled visit, I was having dinner with my daughter and a friend. My phone rang but since the number was not one I recognized, I ignored it. Soon I had two more calls from the same number, so I excused myself and answered the phone. The caller identified himself as a police officer and asked if I knew of a Patricia Bryan. He said he was calling to inform me they found her dead in her bed at home. They saw my number on her refrigerator, the only contact number they could find. I remembered making a home visit a year or so after Mr. Bryan was first discharged from the hospital. I had written my number on a paper and placed it under a magnet on their fridge, inviting them to call me if they needed anything. They never took advantage of it.

Not being a family member, I could not get any more infor-

mation from the police officer. He asked if I knew of any next of
kin so I gave him the niece's name, but I did not have her
number at that time. I did ask him to have Angie call me. I
heard from her less than an hour later. Apparently, her aunt
simply did not wake up from her sleep. We may never know
what happened; we can speculate, but that does not matter.

What mattered was that in a span of less than a year, I lost
my relationship with two wonderful human beings. Again, I
grappled with varied emotions. *Should I have been more atten-
tive? Should I have seen her earlier? What if...?*

I could choose to be riddled with guilt or I can continue to
use these occurrences as stepping stones in my journey and
growth in life. I have to believe that I can only do my best,
intentionally avoid doing wrong, and then trust in what faith
and destiny holds.

What matters—and what I value still today—is the relationship I had with Mr. and Mrs. Bryan. They helped me form a
connection and a sense of community. We developed a sense of
belonging which affirmed the meaning I find in my work. From
such a web of relationships and connections with other people,
we draw our strength, meaning and develop resilience. Such
relationships with our patients promote our own well-being,
both as physicians and people.

ANGIE INVITED me to speak at Patricia's memorial service. I
did, offering gratitude for being blessed with the wonderful
relationship of knowing my patient and his wife. I still have
their photographs prominently displayed on my relationship
board in my office, reminders of beautiful relationships and
gifts that keep on giving. Angie and I remain friends.

And to think, my authentic relationship with the Bryans
began when I had the courage to be vulnerable and humble in
admitting my mistake with his antibiotic and because they had

hearts willing to forgive me. I am amazed at how our experiences will guide our future. Years later, I had a chance to share my hindsight about the value of owning my errors.

———

*Too often we underestimate the power of a touch, a smile, a kind word, a listening ear, an honest compliment, or the smallest act of caring, all of which have the potential to turn a life around.*

LEO BUSCAGLIA

# 14 CAPITOL HILL

*Try not to become a person of success but rather a person of value.*

ALBERT EINSTEIN

IT WAS my first time for Doctors' Day on the Hill in Nashville, where every spring a group of physicians are offered a chance to speak briefly with our state representatives and senators. It's a day to advocate for the needs of our patients and the health system and for legislators to voice appreciation for our care to the community.

In 2010 I was one of ten physicians in Chattanooga chosen by their patients to receive a Doctors' Day award from the Chattanooga Hamilton Medical Society. At the award function, I heard about this chance to speak with state legislators, which the medical society sponsored and made available for physicians and their learners. I decided to go and take a group of residents with me, as I have done every year since then.

The day began with a security check at the state capitol and an agenda of the packed schedule in our hands. Fortunately, we had a knowledgeable, organized, and experienced team leader in the CEO of the medical society. Our role was to educate the leaders representing various constituents regarding the facts behind the important bills on the floor related to health care and its delivery. We had been debriefed and educated with pertinent talking points ahead of time. All this was new, eye-opening, and important. I soaked in the experience.

## Questioning Ethics

At one juncture, a state senator stood and read to us from a letter written by a constituent describing their dissatisfaction with the care received during a recent hospital stay. No details were shared, but the apex erupted in two stunning questions: "Do doctors have a conscience?" and "Is the almighty dollar the carrot?" I felt as if I had been knocked off my feet. The thought had never before crossed my mind that we physicians, who I see as part of a noble profession, are often viewed by the public as being enticed only by money.

Was I naïve? Surely, they knew the reasons we chose this profession were altruistic, so how did they come to this conclusion? This statement stayed with me for quite a while, evoking emotions of surprise, anger, disappointment, sadness, and then a realization of my own belief that perceptions become reality! *If we are perceived this way, we have some part to contribute! What caused this public perception, and how can we undo this?*

It was an aha moment. These questions revealed a perspective completely contradictory from my personal experience in medicine and from that of the learners I taught and trained. I have always valued my profession as one of utmost morality. The author of the letter, however, exposed another side of medical care that demanded my attention. It reaffirmed to me that the practice of medicine was no longer limited to only the patient-physician interaction for clinical care.

We as physicians needed to step up—we needed to be advocates for our patients and profession, possess business acumen, and be transformational leaders. We needed knowledge and training ourselves and to provide the same for our learners if we wanted to ensure this professional nobility. We needed to be at the table when health care policies were being made.

Coming down from the Hill, sitting on the bus, I pondered these questions: *How could I serve to make this difference? What could I and we do?* I definitely needed to educate myself even more by being involved and showing up at meetings. As an educator, I needed to offer such knowledge and opportunities to my learners.

## Sharing Hindsight

Just a few weeks after my experience on Capitol Hill, one late afternoon, a young resident I'll call Stacey came to visit me, clearly in obvious distress. I have an open-door policy, so it is not uncommon for residents and medical students to knock at my door. Stacey often stopped by my office, sometimes to share about an interesting patient she was caring for, other times for career advice or even to share a new recipe or workout routine she had tried.

This day she did not seem herself. Her face did not have her usual big beaming smile. She looked concerned.

"Dr. Panda, do you have a minute?" she asked as she knocked. I looked up from what I was doing, pulled an empty chair closer, and motioned for her to come in. She did, shutting the door behind her. After a minute or two of silence, she spoke, her head still down. "Dr. Panda, I think I made a mistake."

I felt relief. Different thoughts had been racing through my mind: Was she ill? Had she received some bad news?

"I accidently gave Mr. Y the wrong medicine. I had written it correctly, but my handwriting was not clear. The patient is doing okay. He only got two doses, but I feel horrible. What if he had died?"

Illegible handwriting is a common cause for medication errors, which is one thing electronic medical records promises to eliminate (electronic records started at our institution in 2017). My students and residents used to joke about my poor penmanship. I would share that when I was in second grade, I failed handwriting. My mother made me write a page of English and a page of Hindi every day to make my penmanship more legible. I joke with my residents, "If you want an example of horrible handwriting, look at mine. This is what *not* to do."

I had worked with Stacey over the two and a half years of her training. I was always impressed by her attention to detail, her fund of knowledge, and her capacity for compassionate patient-focused care. This mistake was definitely an aberration. I felt her guilt and remorse.

"Stacey, thank you for coming to tell me. I can tell this has been difficult for you."

She shared more details of the patient's hospital course. "I want to let the family know and say I am sorry, but I don't know how. I'm scared. They will never want me to take care of him or anyone. What if they sue me?"

As she asked these questions, tears rolled down her face. My heart felt pained to see her struggle with the tension of wanting to do the right thing and fear of the consequences.

"The patient did recover and became well with no adverse consequences," Stacey continued. "But I didn't mean to harm him!" As she related her anxiety, it was obvious my distraught resident wanted to know not only how she could do better, but how she might apologize to the patient and family. I was truly touched and impressed at her honesty, her desire to do the right thing. The patient's outcome was not impacted by her mistake. She could decide not to say anything—but she wanted to do what she knew was right.

I shared my own personal error of prescribing the wrong antibiotic for Mr. Bryan, which led to some hearing loss. I described my emotions of fear and anxiety similar to hers, as well as my relief when I talked to Mr. Bryan and his wife. I also shared their understanding and our continued relationship in spite of my mistake.

We spent a while speaking about the issue, her own unease, her intentions, and potential consequences. I educated her on the hospital policy regarding errors, disclosure, and apology. She understood and acknowledged the process. We rehearsed the conversation she could have with her patient. I offered to be present if she wanted. Stacey wanted to be by herself when she delivered her disclosure and apology.

Soon after her meeting with the family and patient that evening, Stacey came returned with an update.

"I did it! Everything's okay."

The relief in her voice was obvious, the look on her face was one of joy. She told me how the patient and family expressed appreciation for her honesty. There were no angry accusations, only acceptance and gratitude.

"I'm proud of you, Stacey." I applauded her for her courage to do the right thing. We talked about the role of error in empathy-based medicine and the overall care of the patient. I invited her to think about sharing her story, if and when she felt ready, as an inspiration and educational opportunity for others.

I HAD BEEN INFURIATED when listening to the legislator reading the patient's letter on Capitol Hill. Then this young distraught physician chose to do the right thing. I felt relieved. It gave me faith that honor still exists in our medical profession.

What did this experience do for me? I now had clear

answers for those poignant questions on the Hill. When Stacey came to me so upset about her error, I made a conscious decision as an educator, mentor, and teacher: I chose to role-model the process of identifying with the agitated feelings of a vulnerable patient undergoing treatment. When we physicians take the time to do that with one person, with full presence, then we might be able to advance slowly but surely toward improving society's perception of health care.

I had been practicing medicine in the US for a decade and became a citizen in 1999, but until that day in 2010 I did not begin to understand how the system truly can or cannot work. On that influential day, I realized how important it was for those of us in health care to be involved in policymaking, at least at the state level if not nationally. We can make a positive contribution to the complex and unique form of government known as Democracy.

I also realized, though, that it's not always possible to effect policy change in our health care institutions, even when we hold positions of power in our departments. Other factors are often at play that we cannot control. And that's when we have to decide where to stand in our values.

———

*Even the smallest act of caring for another person is like a drop of water—it will make ripples throughout the entire pond.*

JESSY AND BRYAN MATTEO

# 15 THE MEASURE OF A LIFE

*One's life has value so long as one attributes value to the life of others.*

SIMONE DE BEAUVOIR

METRICS. Charts. Graphs. Spreadsheets. Neat numbers shown in a colorful, visually appealing display to illustrate multi-layered, quantity-based outcomes. These are the standards to which medical care professionals are bound each and every day across disciplines, specialties, and ranks throughout the compensation scale. These numbers define how we measure success in today's fiercely competitive quest for a coveted position on the "A" list of hospitals.

When I was the chair of the department of internal medicine, part of my job was to review the monthly spreadsheets provided by the hospital that chart Relative Value Units (RVUs) of each of the faculty in the department, including mine. Relative value units are a measure of value used in the United States Medicare reimbursement formula for physician services.

One day while heavily engaged in this task of reviewing an

RVU spreadsheet, my inpatient-ward team and I were called to the emergency room to attend a Caucasian woman in her mid-50s for fluid in the abdomen. I'll call her Ms. J. As was customary, the resident with the team of interns and students went to see the patient first before presenting and evaluating the patient with the physician preceptor. They paged me about thirty minutes later, informing me that they were ready to present the patient to me. I headed to the ER. The presentation began with, "This patient is a frequent flyer to various neighborhood emergency rooms." Apparently, Ms. J had visited multiple emergency rooms over the past six to eight weeks for the same complaints. Each time she was treated appropriately for her acute symptoms by having the fluid removed for relief and discharged her with instructions to follow up with her primary care physician.

Over the years my experience has taught me to have my radar up when I hear the term "frequent flyer." For one thing (though I am guilty of using this terminology too), I feel it somehow implies a less than desirable character trait of the patient, and second, there is often a need for deeper probing about the reasons for repeat visits. This time was no different. That alert signal remained on as I listened to the team describe the patient's history.

Ms. J had come to our emergency room because her belly was swollen and it was getting difficult for her to breathe. She lay propped up on the stretcher, her swollen belly obvious from the mid-section bump in the sheet covering her. Ms. J looked uncomfortable and tired, with sunken cheeks and eyes, and her shallow breaths indicated her difficulty breathing. Review of the multiple prior records indicated an assumption that the woman's condition directly resulted from a lifestyle of excessively drinking alcohol, which causes liver damage and failure that leads to the fluid build-up.

Her son and daughter, who looked to be in their late twenties to early thirties, stood by her side. The daughter was stroking her mother's brow with one hand, the other hand clasping her mother's. She too appeared tired and concerned. The son was pacing the room, looking frustrated, agitated, and restless. He stopped as I entered with the team and gave my extended hand a cursory shake, then asked, "Can you tell us why my mother is so sick? We've seen many doctors, but she keeps getting worse!"

I reassured him that I would do my best, that I needed to ask a few more questions and examine his mother. I proceeded to introduce myself to my patient and her daughter. I began the ritual of taking a detailed history, something I was taught very early in my first year of medical school in India, always take your *own* history and perform your *own* examination of your patient. The daughter and son watched, corroborating their mother's responses or answering for her. My team had done a good job. I got similar facts as theirs.

And then I asked about personal social habits. "Ms. J, have you ever smoked tobacco or anything else? Do you consume alcohol? If so, how much for how long?" As I asked this series of questions, I could see the pain in my patient's eyes.

"Yes, I drink to help me sleep and get over the pain, but I promise, doctor, I only started drinking every day since the last six or eight weeks. Before that I would have a beer or two only once every three to six months. Now I drink wine or liquor, but I still cannot get rid of the pain in my back. I promise you, doctor, I'm not lying. Please believe me." Her son and daughter were nodding their heads in agreement. My patient was telling the truth. Her eyes spoke the truth, and I believed her.

I told Ms. J that I believed her as I held her other hand. I knew I had to get her comfortable first. We needed to get the fluid off her belly to improve her breathing. She and her children agreed. I assured them that I would review all the tests thus far and return to share what I learned and to explain the further plan of care.

As a team we thanked the son and daughter for helping us understand their mother's medical history. We acknowledged their concern. I left the room after my team and the son followed me, asking, "Doctor, will my mother be all right? We have been dealing with this for almost two months. She seems to be getting worse. Please help us. We have been to so many places. They remove the fluid, she feels better for a few hours, but then it builds up again."

"Has she been seen by her primary care physician?" I asked.

"No, doctor," he replied, "My sister and I have to work. The primary care doctor who was assigned is far away, and we cannot miss any more work." There was a sense of desperation in his voice. "Also, will you be able to sign my FMLA papers? I have missed so many days of work."

I promised that I would help him with his papers and, more immediately, help him understand why his mother was sick as soon as I had a better understanding of her condition. My team and I made arrangements for our patient to have her procedure emergently.

## Detective Work

Something about the perfunctory diagnosis Ms. J carried was disturbing. Six to eight weeks of heavy drinking should not lead to liver failure. There had to be another reason. I often tell my students that part of presence as a physician comes from tuning into their own instincts. I say, "What is your gut telling you about the patient's story? You must listen to your patient's story and to your gut."

It was late evening when I completed my rounds on three remaining patients. My team left to complete their notes while the intern caring for our patient and I researched Ms. J's history some more. Systematically I thumbed through all the paper records that had been sent with the patient summarizing her emergency room visits in the past two weeks. I then started scrolling through all the information available in our electronic records. I navigated the mouse on the desktop in the emergency room, my intern and I hunting for some clues. I spoke out aloud, interpreting various laboratory results, using this as a teaching opportunity. I ran through the differential diagnosis of the causes of fluid buildup in the belly, emphasizing the need to rule out gynecological causes like tumors of the ovary.

"Let's see if she has had any imaging of her abdomen or pelvis," I said. Finding none in the records we had and having confirmed during the history-taking that our patient had not had pelvic surgery, we decided to get a stat imaging study to see if we could uncover any cause of fluid buildup related to her ovaries. As I reviewed the results about an hour later, my worst fears were proven correct. Ms. J had a large growth on one of her ovaries with multiple smaller tumors in her lungs, liver, and belly lining. These could explain her fluid buildup and unrelenting back pain. She was suffering the late-stage complications of ovarian cancer. She was terminally ill and quite literally on her deathbed.

Unfortunately, when Ms. J arrived in the emergency room, she probably had been stereotyped. Perhaps her presentation with intractable fluid in her abdomen coupled with her being a frequent flyer had led to this assumption. Such stereotyping is a type of cognitive bias that leads to premature closure, or a failure to stop and ask, "What else could it be?"

## Bedside Manners

We reconvened our team and shared our conclusions. It was time to break the news to Ms. J and her children. My senior resident and I decided to be the ones to share our findings. He knelt by her bed to be in eye contact, while I sat on her bed and held her hand. The children stood by, their concern and anticipation visible through their facial expressions.

The exact words of my resident are gone from memory, but he kindly explained what we saw in the imaging and that Ms. J was in the end stages of ovarian cancer, which was causing the fluid buildup and swelling of her belly.

Ms. J just looked at us and her children, and she nodded without saying a word. Her grip on my hand remained tight. Her daughter burst into tears. Her son shook his head, his voice loud and angry, "How long has this been going on? What can be done? We are ready to take her to any specialist."

The daughter could see her mother, despite her silence, was becoming disturbed by their emotional reactions. She asked her brother to take his concerns outside the room.

"Why don't we step out into the hall and I can explain in more detail, while we let your mother rest," I suggested. My resident followed, and the three of us sat down on some chairs in a quiet place a few feet away from his mother's room. Slowly my resident and I shared details about the extent of her illness, the complications affecting her other organs. I assured Ms. J's son that I would get a cancer specialist to see his mother for another opinion, which he appreciated. As the reality unfolded, his eyes welled up with tears too. We were able to get the on-call oncology team to see the patient within the hour. Their conclusions and discussions confirmed our patient's diagnosis of terminal ovarian cancer.

I felt that Ms. J knew she was very sick, but she had not been ready to die. Everything was happening too rapidly, especially for the children. They went from not knowing what was going on, to finding out about the cancer, to holding out hope of their mother getting better with treatment. Instead, within a matter of hours, they needed to come to terms that their mother was dying.

## Time Well Spent

I made the choice to be with these family members, spending hours holding hands with Ms. J's son and daughter, guiding them through the stages of grief. I assured them I would make sure that their mother would be comfortable, that we would do everything to ease her physical suffering, even if that meant she would be less able to continue interacting with them. They were relieved to hear that. With their permission I called the chaplain to assist us all as together we experienced this journey of saying goodbye.

My team could not stay, but were required to leave because they were bound by the regulatory duty hours. At that moment I was focused on tending to the family's emotions, but later I realized that I was also holding my own tension about being held to RVUs. The standard relative value unit requirement rewards seeing more patients and has no method to accurately account for the prolonged time spent consoling and supporting patients and their families. I stayed anyway.

Ms. J died in the early hours after midnight with her son and daughter by her side.

I left the room, my heart and body heavy with varied emotions, physical and emotional exhaustion. I was sad at the outcome, yet thankful for trying to help the best we could. And I was angry. I was not sure exactly why I was angry. I ran through a litany of my own internal diagnostic questions. *Was it at the outcome, my inability to do more, or was it at the system that is difficult for patients to navigate? What if she had been able to see her primary care physician early on when her symptoms began? What if Ms. J had had easy access to routine preventive care? What if...?*

I knew that as advanced as her disease was, it would still have been terminal eight weeks ago. My rational mind also reminded me that I was wrong to blame this event entirely on a broken system. It is much more complex and convoluted, with each stakeholder being responsible—physicians, patients, and the system alike. But at this moment, my inner emotional voice was much louder than my rational one!

The more I thought about my reaction, the angrier I grew—mostly at my own powerlessness. I felt powerless despite my role as the department chair of internal medicine. I was not able to effectively justify the case for RVUs being an accurate measure of physician value, especially in an academic teaching setting. I had failed myself and my department faculty.

## What is a Relative Value Unit?

RVUs are an archaic attribute giving a numerical value to the work done by a physician based on time and acuity of illness. Hospitals look at work production of a physician often based purely on RVU. Many institutions incentivize positions financially over and above the RVU allocated. For instance, your job description says if you're hired at this level, you have to make so many RVUs per day, such as laying hands on ten patients with certain illnesses.

What you enter depends on the number of diagnoses. A patient may have hypertension and stroke and kidney failure and heart failure, but comes in with just gallstones. You did not take care of anything but gallstones that day, but if you document in such a way that it appears you've taken care of all the sicknesses, you may make more RVUs than your actual work entailed. It requires true integrity and honesty from everybody involved.

Unfortunately, this metric doesn't account for anything else except what is documented by the physician or team taking care of the patient.

Can RVUs be inaccurate, intentionally or unintentionally? Yes. Has it really happened? Yes, I've experienced it myself. I was present when a close relative was admitted to the hospital and examined. After gaining my relative's permission, I asked the compliance officer and the chief nursing officer to see her records. I looked at the physician's detailed description of what had been performed on my relative as a history and physical. I knew that not even one-tenth of what was documented had been done. That particular physician had not laid hands on the patient. While this is one personal experience, I have heard many similar accounts from colleagues and friends. This is just one of the ways that the RVU is truly faulty.

If RVU becomes the largest carrot dangled in front of physicians, where does quality of patient relationships go? You can't get paid for time spent getting to know your patients, *really* knowing about them beyond their illness, their life with and without the context of their illness. But such time is invaluable. Quantity over quality, I feel, is the biggest flaw of RVUs.

While there are metrics for quality of care, the quality of patient/physician relationships is part of care but rarely recognized or incentivized. Quality of meaningful relationships is never measured, but it could be. You can capture patient perceptions of physician empathy with an empathy scale or compassion scale, or capture qualitative data by gathering patient stories and testimonials. If you really want to measure, there's data for everything.

So where in the RVU can we include a value for the *true* R, the *Relationship* Value Unit? Where is the worth of human touch shown on a spreadsheet? How is our time to role-model the grieving process turned into a quantifiable unit of success? Where does emotional or spiritual health fit into the metrics? In academic settings, the vital time spent on the task of education itself is often overlooked in this physician effectiveness and value equation. Because such values are not part of currently available computer programs, in most North American culture they are not recognized at all.

Bringing Back the R

One of the initiatives I'm championing now, almost a decade later, is called "Bringing Back the R in RVU—Relationship Value Unit." The goal is to create a culture that invites and permits the development of relationships and explores how these relationships impact the various metrics on the current dashboard (such as patient satisfaction, quality of care, and physician satisfaction). Subtle gauges for measurement could be measuring physician engagement, staff retention and recruitment, patient adherence, and patient feedback. Another important element is creating a community of physicians who believe in a shared covenant of holistic patient care and colleague care, who agree that our work is not a competition of one against the other, and who trust that we are all in this together.

Incentivizing people for building relationships and for education itself would mean giving a relationship value unit, an education value unit, and an empathy value unit the same weight as the relative value unit. They would all count toward an incentive.

Relationships are not only important between physician and patient. Relationships must start with a relationship with our self (which requires internal reflection) and a relationship with our colleagues (which requires trust building). Good relationships with our stakeholders are vital, such as hospital administrators and leaders who are not practicing clinicians. Even in non-teaching hospitals, oftentimes it appears that the C-Suite administrative leaders are the people in suits who work eight to five while they run a 24/7 hospital. They are seldom present in the middle of the night when there's minimal staff and things often go wrong. They appear to make judgments and decisions for, not with, the people who have their boots on the ground. Authentic relationships between physicians and "the suits" would lead to better decisions for patients and staff. Would not a shared relationship with shared decision-making result in win-win situations?

I feel that the accountability pendulum has swung too far. I find myself questioning with strong sentiments the audacity of the decision-makers to ask for data to make a case for something that is the very essence of humaneness. The sacredness and value of the patient/physician relationship developed over time has been swept away, leaving in its place a cold, impersonal computer screen. The importance of evaluations, ratings, and performance measurements geared toward quantity of measures distract from the value and quality of each human life. Various quantitative inhuman measures have twisted the Hippocratic Oath into a business model which does great harm to both medical care professionals and to their patients. To define success, we of course must require monitors and measures. And of course, I need to be accountable too! As a physician and leader, I too am a key stakeholder in the system. Did I do my part?

Physicians also need to take ownership in advocating for change to this RVU paradigm. We need to permit, invite, and ensure time to develop and nurture relationships. Our engagement will promote partnerships between physicians and the stakeholders, allowing for shared decision-making around an aligned mission and vision. Our voices belong alongside the C-Suite executives. Patients' voices also belong in the conversation because their important opinions could contribute to the change process, and patients can affirm to other stakeholders the value of their physicians.

## The Final Straw

Just as we diagnose our patients, diagnosing our learners is equally paramount. Learners come with different educational foundations and knowledge bases, individual strengths and needs. Further, our team comprises learners at different levels of training, third- and fourth-year medical students, residents in their first and second and third years. Often, we have a pharmacy student and physician assistant students on the team too. We need to diagnose these diverse learning needs of our learners and tailor our teaching and the educational modalities. This step requires an intentional investment, which is time consuming. Unfortunately, often that is compromised for the volume pressures, the predictor of RVUs, time being the limiting constant.

I was overwhelmed by the pressure. The tension of volume versus value, service versus education, was one that kept me awake at night. As faculty, we all want to be good educators, but that requires time and permission to be effective.

As their department chair, I was unable to give the faculty an environment for doing their work in a way that felt satisfying and meaningful for them.

I remember the advice of a dear and seasoned mentor. I had sought his wisdom after I was offered the job as chair of the department of medicine. He said, "Mukta you will have to become thick-skinned. People will knock on your door often, but not to thank you, only to complain or ask for more money. Further, you will not be paid for the many sleepless nights you will face!" How correct he was!

It was during the same time period while I was caring for Ms. J that this RVU issue was especially weighing heavily on my mind. The budget cycle was fast approaching, and I had many discussions with the dean about my conundrum and tension. The financing and funding of health care is truly complex, and I was having difficulty aligning the ideal with the reality. However, my tensions were not unique. The dean was very understanding. Compromises were needed.

My scheduled meeting with the leadership to review the

coming academic year's budget and expectations was just a few days after the emotional encounter with Ms. J and her children, and her death. At the meeting I shared yet again my concerns about faculty dissatisfaction and educational compromise and my overwhelming tension about RVUs. "I don't know how to bridge this disagreement," I said in despondency.

"Mukta, unfortunately we don't have another choice."

"I don't know if I can continue like this. I don't think I'm the best person for the job anymore." There it was, I finally spoke out loud what I had ruminated over many times in my sleepless nights.

## More Than One Reason

I was beginning to see that it was time to step down as chair of the department of medicine. It was a complicated decision.

Before that day I had felt the push from other quarters to step down: subtle but immensely palpable discriminations, pay inequalities, and bullying, to name a few. But Ms. J's life—and death—counted in too many immeasurable ways, and feeling the agony of "volume over value" that night was my final straw.

In addition, I had been facing another ongoing tension. I was under pressure to preferably recruit US graduates for our department and not consider non-US medical graduates. I often felt expected to allow a slightly lower recruitment criteria and that felt not only hypocritical, but too much to shoulder.

I realized this pressure was not a matter of what was right or wrong. It was not plain and simple, not black or white. These issues are driven by many factors, many decisions, at levels beyond my understanding. I realized, however, that I could no longer align myself with the organization's mission while maintaining my professional ethics. Sensing and hoping there was another, better way to serve, I did not yet hold a clear vision of how to proceed. I knew only that I needed to voice my decision with courage—after all, resigning my position entailed significant financial, professional, emotional, and personal risk.

I understood that the environment at my institution was not unique; other institutions across the nation had similar policies. The pressures and motives were many and varied, which I'm sure I did not fully comprehend. Leadership lenses were different. Each was only doing what they felt to be right from their viewpoint. I also was mindful that my lens was influenced and probably biased by my varied experiences across the globe.

I knew I had to resign as chair because I needed the change. I believe a good leader needs to know how to *leave* well (not just *lead* well) and, more importantly, a good leader needs to know *when* to leave. Times had changed, and I felt that I was in the minority yet again, this time as an academician. Each person was fulfilling their mission; each had the mission of providing the best patient care as their covenant. We disagreed on the best way to do so. However, now that I recognized my feelings, staying in my position of department chair felt wrong, even hypocritical.

"I think you need to find someone else for this position," I said, after sharing my feelings and concerns.

"What do you mean, Mukta? What else might you do here? What would you like to do?"

"My passion is in education and patient care," I said.

"Would you consider working with medical students?"

Frankly speaking, while I had explored other options and had unsolicited offers from colleagues in other institutions, I felt an allegiance to the place where I trained. I had taken a risk letting the leadership know that they needed to find someone else for my position. But I felt able to share my true concerns. Over the years our communication was authentic and felt safe.

## Liberating My Voice

Immediately following the determination to go ahead and step down as department chair, I felt liberated and even more energized to continue the work. I began a new position as assistant dean for medical student education, which offered me a way to be more truly aligned to my core values. It felt right in my soul. The burden had been lifted. I could now speak forth more authentically and stand alongside the C-Suite and educational leaders who did embrace and walk the mission. This was not the first time I had shared my frustration with the system, but now I spoke from firmer, more confident ground.

This pure gift of grace and the events leading up to it did much for my faith. As the wisdom saying goes, when God closes one door, he always opens another. Sometimes I can only look up, smile, and say thank you. I am taking small steps along the way, moving through the door in trust. Sometimes our life experience is very scary and we don't yet have the voice or language to express ourselves, but by telling our stories and encouraging others to do the same, we build a community. That we are all in this life together is the most important realization of all.

*Life lived under the performance principle makes us slaves to insecurity and anxiety, constantly comparing ourselves to others, struggling to reach a level of achievement which always eludes us. Life seen as "gift," as grace, can set us free. Once you know you are loved unconditionally by God, there is such freedom.*

GEOFFREY TRISTRAM, SSJE

# 16 THE GOOD PHYSICIAN

*High technology will always be complementary to human
touch; without human touch it is just deadweight, like
archives, fossils, and museum specimens.*

SHYAM PARASHAR

EVER SINCE THE fateful day when I walked through the
tunnel joining our office building to the parking lot and discovered the limp, lifeless form of my friend and colleague, I have
wrestled with the meaning and value of our work, our lives,
and our calling as physicians. My friend ended his very fruitful
life in despair, having been systematically and relentlessly
devalued over the years by the very career to which he had
given his heart, mind, body, and soul.

This good physician moved through his days at the hospital
with a warm, open smile for everyone, all the while struggling
in a health care system that is often unwelcoming to solo practitioners. In the early 2000s, he enjoyed a stable practice and was
an inspiration to those of us who encountered him each day.
His dedication and work ethic were clear for all to see. He

always wore a short white coat, a white shirt, and khaki pants. That was his uniform. Behind his spectacles, he had kind blue eyes. A dermatologist, he had great skin. Disciplined, highly observant, ethical in large and small matters, this man possessed an immense desire for lifelong learning. His enthusiasm was contagious. He took great pleasure in spontaneously sharing his knowledge and findings.

I knew him as a physician since 1995, and from 2007 I knew him as a colleague when I became chair of the department of medicine and he was a faculty member. Our offices were across the street from the hospital. I was on the second floor and he was in private practice on the fourth floor where he was leasing space from the hospital. A tunnel connects the hospital and office buildings. Our paths would cross in the tunnel, and he would always take time to wish me well, and I would wish him well in return. Having passed each other several times one day, he noticed a spot on my cheek.

"Mukta, I need to take a look at that."

"Sure, doctor," I said, but I didn't make an appointment.

A few weeks later he saw me again and said, "When are you coming to see me?" It would take several more kind prompts before I finally heeded his concern.

HIS OFFICE WAS full of stories. He still preferred paper charts to electronic medical records. His nurse greeted me with a warm smile; she had been with him for over fifteen years. He proudly showed me a photograph of himself with two of his three sons and his son-in-law on the golf course at the Masters in Augusta. This was a gift of love to him from all his children and their families. His shelves held photos of patients and exotic places around the world. Potted orchids of different hues were all over his office.

During my appointment, he explained about my skin lesion

and took time taking my full medical history. The good physician gave me detailed instructions about why I needed to get it taken care of, explaining the importance of the skin as an organ. He emphasized the importance of sunscreen.

"I love growing orchids," he said, "but I garden before the sun comes up or after it sets. Even then, I always wear sunscreen." His skin was immaculate even though he was seventy-six years old.

"I know about sunscreen now in America," I said, "but I never grew up with sunscreen in India." I enjoyed speaking with him. You could easily spend an hour or more in his company because he had so much to talk about. That appointment really began our relationship. He helped me take care of that lesion, which could have been precancerous.

Only one thing seemed almost at odds with his kindness and compassion. That was his attachment to his designated parking space next to our office building. Nobody was allowed to park in his spot, even if it was empty. One time, my daughter parked there for a few minutes to briefly visit me. He left a stern sticky note on her windshield. It said something like, "This spot is reserved. Do not park here. Please move the vehicle immediately." That was his one pet peeve. We respected it. I took him an orchid as a peace offering and we laughed about it afterwards.

AROUND 2015 THERE was a lot of change within the organization, including a reengineering of the building spaces for physicians and patients. I had made my decision to step down as department chair and was moving into the dean's office. It was autumn and we were all busy moving.

One Wednesday afternoon he stopped by my office. I was surrounded by boxes. "Mukta, I need to know what to do," he said. "They're asking me to leave my office. I need to work and take care of my wife." He'd brought a big portfolio of photos he had prepared for teaching. "Look, I want to teach. I have all this teaching material." He hated technology, but had gotten a computer and trained himself to make PowerPoint presentations, converting his old slides into PowerPoints. "I want to continue doing this."

"Who is *they*?" I asked him.

"I don't know. I got an email from the hospital telling me to move."

"Look, I'm moving too. This is an institution-wide change. Have you thought about joining the hospital practice?"

"Yes, but you know how I like my way of working. I can't see fifteen to twenty patients in four hours," he said. "I like to spend time with my patients."

"I don't know what to do about that. I am not in a position of authority anymore. I am leaving myself. But I can definitely try to help get you involved in teaching the students. We'll have to talk to the university leadership about that."

"I don't even know who that would be," he said.

"Look, let's get an appointment for you with the university leadership." I walked with him downstairs to the medical education office, where he made an appointment for that Friday. I found out later they did have the meeting and that it went okay.

IT WAS a busy week for me, packing up my office and balancing my physician duties with family time. My daughter and her husband were in Chattanooga visiting. That Sunday, they had a six-a.m. flight back to New York City, so I dropped them off at the airport and went to the office early.

I remember it was a crisp Sunday morning, November 15, 2015. I worked until about 9:30 a.m. and decided that was enough—I would go home and enjoy the rest of my weekend. I walked out the sliding glass door toward the parking lot and saw a figure wearing a hoody and gloves, as if they'd gone for a long run and were sitting on the ground stretching forward to touch their toes. Nobody else was around. I stopped short and yelled out, "Hello, are you okay? Hello?" No movement. I rushed back into my office and called security, "I need some help out there." I walked back out to the sliding glass door and still saw no movement. I waited. The police car drove up and I began to approach them outside. They signaled to me to wait, saying "There's blood all around." I went slowly around the side of the policemen who were gathered around the body. By this time the Emergency Medical Services Ambulance had arrived. I just knew in my gut it was my friend. The EMTs started cardiopulmonary resuscitation immediately, and he was rushed to the emergency room.

As I watched, I understood the grim prognosis. I was being asked a lot of questions by the hospital administrator on call and the police. I shared what I knew. Truly, I was in a state of shock and not sure what I needed to do. I tried calling the dean but he didn't answer. Then I called the chief financial analyst. "It's Dr. ___. I hope he has not hurt himself." Those were my words, because we just didn't know. I couldn't help thinking that he had tried to hurt himself.

I recognized another colleague's car in the same parking lot, which hadn't been there when I arrived. I called her. "Did you see anything when you came to work?" She said "No," so we knew it had happened in the last thirty minutes.

Thoughts flashed through my head. *What if I had come outside earlier? What if, what if, what if...* I just couldn't think anymore so I got into my car and went home. I knew the best thing I could do was to leave the scene and try to unpack in my mind what had happened. At home I told my parents. I was dumbstruck. I couldn't tell anybody else because of the police investigation. That evening the hospital CEO called with a few questions. There wasn't much to say.

## What Ifs

When a tragic death happens like this, we want to know why. Like anyone, I looked for answers. Being in the middle generation, I see a constant battle between Baby Boomers and Millennials. Vocation is everything to the Boomers—they are the breadwinners, hard workers, devoted to their jobs. Younger physicians want quick results and are more efficient with technology. They value their recreation and time with their families. Each generation has so much to teach the other. My colleague and friend, the good physician, was invited to join a hospital practice with very young dermatologists and a four-day work week. He was being asked to fit into a mold—not right or wrong—but one he couldn't align with. To me, it seemed he was holding that tension in a way that was agitating him. He wasn't sure where he belonged anymore. He couldn't keep doing what he knew so well, and he felt like he didn't have the tools or the courage to try something new.

I asked myself, *Should I have had a different conversation with him that day? Was I too busy with my own frustrations, with the change in the direction of the organization's leadership, my decision to step down as chair? Was my lens already biased? When he came to see me that day, what did I miss so I don't miss it in others?*

While I don't have guilt, I went through all the phases of asking "What could I have done more or differently?" and "How can I make sure this never happens again?" I felt anger, asking "Why did we let this happen?" It was not why did *I* let this happen, but more why did *we*. I say this with humility: I never took the blame solely on my shoulders. In part, that's because I already felt so tainted by the toxic work environment, with its constant focus on volume, speed, and productivity over quality, humanity, and building relationships. But also—and this is important—it's a point of self-care to know you can't be solely responsible for a system.

ON MONDAY BACK AT WORK, I heard many different sides of the story and that he had left a note. I heard he had made arrangements for pending payments.

Two things happened after that.

A conversation with a colleague on Monday made me angry. It started with sympathy but quickly turned into dismissiveness. "Mukta, I'm really sorry. I heard what happened."

I was already livid with grief, "I know, but we should have done something."

"I heard he had some problems."

That made me even more livid.

"No," I said. "You know, he came to me recently. He told me he needed to keep working." I shared the many varied reasons my friend, the good physician, had mentioned, the main ones being his passion for his vocation and teaching, his love and care for his patients, and his thirst for lifelong learning.

"Well, I always been told the other shoe can drop at any time," my colleague said. "You have to have reserves."

"Not everyone has that option," I replied, getting more upset. "We spend eight hours of our day working here. We have to look at ourselves and ask ourselves what we could have done. We have to take care of each other, support each other."

"I look for that support outside the hospital," he said.

"Again, not everybody has that luxury." I didn't want to talk anymore. To me, his reaction seemed callous.

He looked at me and said, "Obviously you're upset about it. I hope you take as much time as you want. If you need help, just let us know." I was getting even more furious by this point.

I took a deep breath then and shifted into gratitude. I

looked up to the heavens and said to myself, "It's no coinci-
dence—I don't believe in coincidences, only confirmations."
On that very day, it so happened that I was flying to Chicago for
a symposium on physician well-being hosted by the Accreditation Council for Graduate Medical Education (ACGME). I
would ponder this tragedy there.

## Hazards of the Healing Profession

The impetus for the ACGME symposium had come from the
family of a medical resident named Greg Feldman. If you
search online for his name, you will see that his promising
accolades included being a star student at Harvard Medical
School, volunteering for surgical mission trips to help children
in Rwanda, roles in leadership, a prestigious residency at
Harvard followed by an award-winning surgical fellowship at
Stanford School of Medicine. He had been four months into
another fellowship in Chicago. But in 2010, at the age of thirty-
three, Greg became one of the disproportionate number of
physicians who end their own lives. His family charged the
ACGME to do something about this crisis of physician suicide
and burnout.[1]

A letter from his family posted online reads, "Greg had one
of the brightest personal futures and groundbreaking careers
ahead of him. We believe, however, that the professional experience he endured in the months before he died triggered a
rapid, overpowering unraveling."[2]

The symposium was limited to 100 attendees. We met in
small groups to discuss possible solutions to practical but
complex questions. What could be done to promote resilience?
What would facilitate early identification and recognition of
distressed residents? What efforts would reduce the stigma that
surrounded seeking help? How might we ensure access to care?
How could we intervene to help grieving communities heal?

(The thought of helping a grief-stricken community heal was very close to home.)

The second day, in small groups again, one question became a seed that would begin to grow in my heart. "What would you be able (willing) to commit to do personally/organizationally over the next year?" Was there a way I could go back and effect an organizational culture change?

The symposium was a time for catharsis. Two close friends were there who gave me a safe space to be open and share my frustration, anger, and sadness without feeling like I needed to make a point. It was a gift to have someone to listen to me. I asked for their suggestions about how to approach change in my institution. "How would you even begin to have such conversations with people?"

One possible first step, they suggested, would to be gather a group of residents and colleagues who had the opportunity to work with the good physician and simply allow them to speak.

Being at the symposium was a blessing because it gave me a sense that I could do something positive. I could use this tragic event as an imperative to move things forward. Being there, hearing other stories and the tools other organizations had used, gave me renewed energy, a burning desire, to move institutional change forward. I was invigorated to go back to work and start a well-being committee. People knew I was upset about what had happened to our good physician. Honestly, I didn't care if they thought I was also a victim. I decided I was going to utilize that empathy, because it meant they would listen to me.

## Paying Tribute

The day I returned to work after the symposium, I had a voice message from his wife, who I did not yet know personally. I mustered the courage to call her back, unsure what she might say.

"Dr. Panda, I don't know what to do. He has so much stuff in his office. He always spoke so kindly of you and you helped him. Can you use some of his stuff?"

I had three students going into dermatology, so we walked upstairs and looked through his office together. Throughout his career, he had never failed to go to annual conferences on dermatology at the Mayo Clinic. He had a book from the 1963 Mayo Clinic proceedings. One of my students was going to study dermatology at the Mayo Clinic, so he took that book. I kept a picture of him at a health fair. Then we found lecture notes in a manila envelope. He was so organized. He had created a lecture on skin lesions for the residents, complete with facilitator notes and a PowerPoint. A thought came to me. I immediately called his wife and told her what we had found.

"I'd like to re-give this lecture," I said. "My students will give it in his honor to celebrate him. Would you be willing to let us do that?"

She said yes. My medical students and I planned the event, inviting his family, residents, and colleagues. We delivered his lecture. We celebrated his life with our own stories in his honor.

In some ways that celebration began healing my wound. I had felt I needed to do something. More so, I wanted to celebrate and affirm him as the astute, kind and compassionate physician and educator he was. I wanted him remembered as somebody who had given so much of himself as a human being, as a friend, as a physician, as a teacher, as a community servant. And as a father, a grandfather, and a husband.

## The Trouble with the Triple Aim

We walk through a journey in the health care system that outright devalues non-financial, qualitative, non-normative results in favor of quantitative measures. It's easier to show stakeholders a progression of numbers on spreadsheets. And often by hacking the quality of patient care, there is the added bonus of slashing expenses. The shift to the Triple Aim, [3] introduced in 2007—with three well-intended initial goals of improving the patient care experience, improving population health, and reducing per-capita health care costs—garnered widespread appeal. Sometimes referred to as the Triple Aim, and other times as The Holy Grail, these ambitions may have had unintended consequences, as well-intended experiments often do. The Triple Aim left out one of the major stakeholders —the physicians. What about them? What about understanding what connected physicians' passion to their purpose? While the original three goals were admirable, the population-wide focus on the Triple Aim prevented too many of us from noticing the increasing rates of physician burnout, depression, and suicide.[4]

That over half our physicians nationwide are affected by burnout is a rampant rate of eye-opening proportions. Such an alarming reality in the US is beyond acceptability. Burnout is associated with lower patient satisfaction, reduced health outcomes, and it may increase costs.

In 2016 the Triple Aim was amended with the Quadruple Aim of improving the experience of providing care by bringing back joy and meaning to medicine.[5] But is it too late? Much damage has already occurred. What is the cost of a human life?

My good friend couldn't keep up with the quantity dictate. It destroyed him, along with thousands more physicians that we know of who are suffering immeasurably.

Unlike many other industries with serviceable quantitative

measures, health care cannot be forced into like categories. Does a quantity of a single human life make any sort of sense? An outcome of one human loss is called a tragedy. Outcomes of many human losses are called statistics. Statistics generate celebration for those who process them or are benefitted by them, but we no longer have the luxury of placing peoples' lives on par with a chart full of numbers.

The great stories in health care are about patient/physician relationships. How can a quantitative statistic be measured and celebrated over human connection? We must retrain our focus to celebrate the "who" along with the "what" in reports of improved patient care and population health.

Medical students and residents are asked to write personal statements for their medical school and residency applications, describing why they are answering the vocational call to health care. In their reflection essays, that very element of human contact shows up over and over as the most important theme. These essays speak of our noble intentions to join a vocation of serving, quenching our thirst for making a difference—we speak of connection to our purpose, we speak of personhood. We speak not of power, possessions, or position.

But how do we as educators support and encourage our students' eloquent answers? Do we give our students and residents the proper tools, or make them aware of even a modicum of necessary self-care habits and resources? Seldom.

Conversely, we celebrate those who are able to separate mind, body, and soul. We further equip young men and women with highly developed obsessive-compulsive tendencies. We demand superhuman hours that effectively produce a mass workaholic mentality.

We as educators must take responsibility for this debilitating situation. We are crying for help to teach this invisible or hidden curriculum. If we and those we work with do not recognize the need for returning humanity to our classrooms, then we are in grave danger of becoming nothing more than robots. Evidence shows how physicians lose our sense of purpose very quickly, as early as after the first year of medical school training. Our systems need to be scrutinized. We need to look deeply into ourselves. Are we the role models we want to be?

I wonder if the pendulum shifted too far over to the non-human pole. I often feel that we in health care put on so many protective layers until they hardened into a self-protective yet destructive shell and we're forgetting who we are. Further, we aren't allowed to be human beings because the model we are held to feels dehumanizing. Every human being needs a sacred space where each belongs and can be brave enough to show up authentically. But currently we do not have permission to come to work wholly as ourselves.

What is the solution? We cannot survive if we continue to follow inhumane institutional practices. The calcified layers we've assumed must begin to crack so that we can see the light at the end of the long figurative tunnel. We need the national dialogue already initiated between various stakeholders like the Accreditation Council of Graduate Medical Education, the National Academy of Medicine, the American College of Physicians, the Arnold P. Gold Foundation, the Collaborative for Healing and Renewal in Medicine (CHARM), other leaders, and those with "boots on the ground." We must rediscover our shared covenant and values.

Along with this national discussion, we each need to take it upon ourselves to walk our talk. Remaining true to your values takes courage and practice. Only then will there be a paradigm shift in the prevailing culture of health care.

Conversation Starters

From the ACGME Symposium on Physician Well-Being, I went back to work with some good ideas as a burning platform to make change in my own institution. I reached back out to one of the friends I'd had dinner with at the symposium because she had experience initiating programs for promoting a culture of well-being in health care organizations. She was kind enough to share a draft proposal of what she thought would be a start.

Unfortunately, the time was not right. The institution was not ready then to have an outside consultant and the cost too was prohibitive. After my initial disappointment, I decided to work on my own. I solicited support from kindred partners in the chief nursing officer along with a faculty member in the department of medicine who had expressed interest and was well versed in research methodology.

I started having conversations with the university and hospital leadership. I referred to the recent ACGME mandates to emphasize the urgency. I created a talking sheet with facts. I knew I had to speak the language of the stakeholders. I worked hard on my elevator pitch for when I spoke to the hospital leaders, focusing my conversations to show that physician burnout (or lack of well-being) has an impact on patient care, safety, quality, satisfaction and finances. The focus of conversations with the undergraduate and graduate medical education leadership were educational needs, learner well-being, and the need for a culture of well-being to maintain an optimal clinical and learning environment.[6]

Accreditation needs were germane to both. The conversations always ended with the tragic and moral imperatives, my voice growing stronger and loaded with emotion when I shared this need and the story of our colleague who had died by suicide. I tried initially to remain professional—as in emotionally detached—but it was not possible. After a few attempts, I stopped trying to hide my anger and heartbreak and spoke from my heart.

My urgency to do something to promote a culture of care

that supported authentic relationships was both a blessing and a curse. It was the catalyst that energized me, but the inertia I felt was often frustrating and crippling. It felt like the leadership's general attitude was one of denial. *Yes, of course all this is going on in other organizations, but it's not our problem. It's somebody else's problem. We are okay.* This attitude I realized later on was not unique to us. I had to practice my own teachings: be kind to yourself and trust. But it was not easy!

## Data Talks

The university was an easier sell than the hospital because they could more quickly buy into the importance of investing in the well-being of students and residents. However, the need for well-being of the faculty physicians was a harder sell. The hospital leadership wanted to see the data to prove the problem was real. It was another harsh reminder that data does speak! My colleague from the department of medicine was immensely helpful. Though none of us had protected time or resources, we were committed to take some action to create awareness around this epidemic of physician burnout that we were facing in our institutions. After an extensive review of the literature and with my colleague's help, we came up with a proposal and got approval from our Institutional Review Board. We surveyed all the physicians and residents employed in the hospital and university.

The survey was administered in the late summer and we had our results by early autumn. Our numbers mirrored the national means, showing higher rates of burnout in women compared to their male counterparts, and in residents more than faculty. We also had data for individual departments. We indeed had a problem comparable to the national data at our institution! Armed with the results, I had more conversations with the different stakeholders. I began to get traction from a few people who also believed something needed to be done.

Encouraged by these allied colleagues, I created a wellness memo outlining a need for creating a task force with representation from each department and the hospital leadership. I met individually with the dean of the university, the chief executive officer, chief medical officer, and chief nursing officer of our affiliate hospital to get their buy-in. With their approval, the March 2017 wellness memo was addressed to colleagues, residents, fellows, and students of the University of Tennessee College of Medicine—Chattanooga.[7]

The memo outlined our specific goals and aims to (1) understand and promote physician and trainee engagement and well-being, (2) provide resources for physicians and trainees that help them promote their own well-being, (3) discover personal and organizational approaches to prevent and address physician and trainee distress, and (4) create a workplace culture that is energy replenishing.

In May 2017 we facilitated a one-day offsite organizational retreat with members of the Well-Being Task Force and two leaders who were experienced advocates for physician well-being, one from Vanderbilt and the other from the ACGME. Nearly fifty leaders from all areas of the hospital and university convened at the Chattanoogan Hotel to explore how we would transform our organization to promote well-being. People who didn't often work together were mixed into groups: hospital leaders, university leaders, department heads, nurse managers, residents, medical students. We asked them to imagine that our affiliate hospital had been voted the best place to work for the third or fourth time and a reporter was interviewing them, wanting to know what is so good about it. Armed with flip charts and pens, people dove into the thought exercise. After lunch, we asked, "What needs to happen now in the next four years?" We unpacked the challenges of the previous four years and discussed how we might overcome the barriers to well-being. It became clear we must improve communication, trust, and transparency, increase physician engagement, as well as define and align the often-conflicting missions of clinical care and education.

The ideas generated that day and a shared sense of vision and imperative for change eventually led to the establishment of well-being initiatives. Based on the needs identified during the retreat, the task force met regularly every two to three months. We identified the areas for interventions at each program level and overall as an organization. We looked for the low-hanging fruit such as ways to improve day to day efficiency of work and also personal well-being, such as gym access, yoga classes, reflective sessions, or social events. We could begin to work on these offerings as a department and hospital.

Later, and together with the university, we would look at tougher issues that would require culture change. It wasn't yet safe to discuss issues that can stigmatize physicians, such as mental health and substance abuse. In an article in the *New England Journal of Medicine*, one physician describes this hurdle:

"On my own recovery journey, I have often felt branded, tarnished, and broken in a system that still embroiders a scarlet letter on the chest of anyone with a mental health condition. A system of hoops and barriers detours suffering people away from the help they desperately need—costing some of them their lives."[8]

## Finding Neutral Ground

Culture change was not happening at the pace my passion desired. One thing I did to navigate my own frustrations with the political environment was to realize that I have to be creative. *If I'm not getting traction here, what else do I need to do?* It required reflection. I needed to look beyond my four walls.

Chattanooga is unique. In the city center is the University of Tennessee College of Medicine and the affiliate hospital, and within a five-mile radius we have three health care systems, one large insurance carrier, Blue Cross Blue Shield, and a medical society of physicians. A lot of physicians practice in more than one health care system. While there is healthy competition, there is also substantial collegial trust among a generation of physicians who've known each other for decades.

The medical society is the neutral ground. I resonated with the medical society's cause of service to fight for patients, plus care of patient and physician. I have been involved as a board member and now co-chair of the Wellness Task Force that I started through the Chattanooga-Hamilton County Medical Society.

With the help of the CEO of the medical society, we wrote a grant and created a LifeBridge program so that physicians could receive up to six free sessions with a psychologist without jeopardizing their credentials or licensure. This encourages physicians to seek mental health care before they are in crisis, without fear of being stereotyped or stigmatized and without retribution.

## What Can I Control?

From 2016 to 2017 I had to do a lot of growing up myself and maturing. I learned to tell myself, *You don't have to convince everybody. Walk steady yourself first and let your actions speak louder.* I wanted the administrators to see me as more than a touchy-feely doctor they could roll their eyes around. That's when I learned I had to be kind toward myself. I'd get easily frustrated, saying, "Come on, don't you realize this is something we need?"

I want to normalize the culture of vulnerability because we all face it. Before we come to work, we must show a physical fitness for duty. We fear disclosing any mental or behavioral issues. Why is having an emotional issue such a taboo?

I did a lot of outreach to fuel my own passion in a positive way, but also to create the fire where everybody wants to fuel it for a common good. I had to make a choice and a commitment, asking myself, *What do I have control over*? I had to start small and realize that data speaks. I had to find cheerleaders for my own work and be a cheerleader for others. It took courage to challenge and empower myself and others with continuous reflection...halt...reflection...halt. I invited people I knew to be coaches for each other, enforcing the importance of compassion and care, reinforcing that they must interact in kind and gentle ways. It was also important to celebrate and showcase achievements as a confirmation that we could do this together. Our collective courage led to changing the culture and building a community.

There are days I take five steps forward. Some days I will say, "That was a wonderful meeting." Other days, it feels like I'm taking ten steps backward. I am happy with little cumulative outcomes.

## The Secret to Peace

I once had the opportunity to be in the presence of His Holiness the Dalai Lama. I was fortunate to attend a 2016 meeting called "The World We Make," where he was hosted by the Center for Healthy Minds at the University of Wisconsin–Madison.[9] He was a member of the panel that was responding to questions from the audience. What impressed me most was his genuine simplicity and humility.

One person asked His Holiness what he thought was the secret to world peace. I distinctly remember His Holiness looking down for a long while. He was attired in his customary red-orange robe, this time complemented by a ball cap gifted by his host.

After a silence he looked up and broke into laughter, eyes twinkling. Pointing at the member who had asked the question, he responded (I paraphrase), "I do not have the secret to world peace, you have. You take care of him, he takes care of her, she takes care of him and so on, going down the line of people in the row, and you have world peace."

What a weighty invitation for us all, paradoxically simple yet difficult to achieve, and definitely not intangible!

———

*Peacemaking often involves dismantling entrenched power.*

MARY LOU REDDING

# 17 A HOW TO LIVE CURRICULUM

*Wisdom is not an ACGME competency, but it's undoubtedly a prerequisite for the art of healing. In fact, wisdom may very well be the fundamental trait that characterizes a well-rounded physician, since it encompasses empathy, resilience, comfort with ambiguity, and the capacity to learn from the past.*

SALVATOR MANGIONE, MD
AND MARC J. KAHN, MD

AS WE PRACTICE our journey of being physicians, we are never taught how to really live through the challenges of isolation, tensions, burnout, depression, not to mention the grief when patients die and the loss of colleagues due to suicide. Such challenges are often labeled as the hidden or the invisible curriculum. What is needed is what I call the "How to Live" curriculum. For physicians, that includes also knowing how to live through the moments and aftermath of death.

I once had a third-year medical student, I'll call her Mary, who had just started her clinical rotations. She was bright-eyed and bushy-tailed, so to speak. During Mary's first rotation in the hospital, she was taking care of patients in the ICU. In her first week, a patient she had cared for suffered a cardiac arrest and died.

The usual scenario in an emergent situation with a patient whose heart stops beating is to rush in with your team, initiate resuscitative measures with cardiac compressions, call a Code 99, (cardiac arrest is a Code 99), call for the monitors, and put in a breathing tube if needed. If the resuscitation is unsuccessful after all protocol and experience-driven measures have been attempted, the code is called off, meaning there's nothing more to be done medically. There is still so much commotion. Everybody starts dispersing. Oftentimes when you are the physician on call, it's not a patient you've taken care of. You may go and speak to the family if there is no physician member from the patient's care team around. You call the physician who was responsible for the patient, who takes over the care from there. Then you must go on with the next thing, whether that's to continue seeing the last patient, or go to the emergency room, or go to a lecture.

How do we take time to acknowledge when death happens?

When Mary's patient died, she didn't know what to do or who to turn to. She went into the stairwell and sobbed. This was the first time she faced the death of a patient and she felt responsible for the lost life.

## The Artful Practice of Medicine

Mary kept the moment to herself until six months later when she shared the experience and her feelings with fellow medical students. This group of third and fourth-year medical students were sitting on the floor in a gallery at the Hunter Museum of American Art in Chattanooga, a mile northeast of our hospital campus along the Tennessee River. Ten students were there for a reflective session called the Art of Balance: Care of Patients, Care of Physician, which is part of their medical training.

Reflective sessions at the Hunter Museum have been in the making for about twelve years now. I am so grateful for two partners, Adera Causey, the museum's curator of education, and Laurie Allen, executive director of the Southeast Center for Education in the Arts at the University of Tennessee—Chattanooga. We started it as small pilot project in 2006-2007, but the program fell by the wayside because we had no funding. When I was department chair, the museum sessions were occasionally part of the RRRnR session with residents.

In my role as assistant dean of well-being, I introduced it again and got funding because I was wiser on how to speak the language of stakeholders that aligned it to the mission and mandates of the university and hospital. In fact, the humanities like art and drama and music are increasingly being acknowledged as an antidote to physician burnout, as noted in the April 2019 issue of the Cleveland Clinic Journal of Medicine.[1] Data suggests that students who choose to have extra interactions with the arts and humanities exhibit greater resilience, tolerance for ambiguity, and more of the empathetic traits we desire in physicians.

We now hold three-hour sessions on two afternoons a month at the Hunter Museum. The purpose is to create a sacred, brave space that invites learners and physicians to be present around our daily stresses as we practice medicine, such as time scarcity, fear of failure, politics, power dynamics, compartmentalizing their work life from home life. Some of these students have never worked together. They have classes together in first and second years but in third year they are dispersed into smaller groups by specialties, and in fourth year their sense of isolation is even more pronounced. But these biweekly sessions over two years gives these medical students more of a sense of having a cohort or community support.

There are no white coats or badges. We show up in our casual street clothes, although some attend in their comfortable scrubs.

"This is a time to be present for yourself, to be in conversation with yourself and/or your colleagues. It's a time to intentionally reflect."

I introduce each session, especially when new students are present.

"Put away your journals and pencils. Feel your feet on the ground. Take a few deep breaths."

That day, the students sat on the floor, looking up at an abstract piece of art on the wall titled Charles Biederman, #17, 1977. On a bright blue background there was a diagonal pattern of wood and aluminum squares, literally jutting out in varying three-dimensional lengths of orange, red, purple, turquoise, and blue. The way each shape protruded from the canvas created real shadows on the surface.

The students were not there to understand the history or theory behind Biederman's art, but to let the artwork itself invite them into conversation about their lives at that moment. In past monthly sessions at the museum, we had talked about accepting responsibility for their own fragility and finding their own strength amidst uncertainty. Today we wanted to continue that focus and talk about the balance between strength and weakness.

Honestly, we could have had the same conversation in front of a still-life of fruit, or an Impressionist painting of sail boats at a city park, or by using a poem or a YouTube video. The secret is not found in the style or content of the artwork but in the possibility for students to access a different part of their brains and hearts. In fact, we later sent the medical students out into the gallery to find even more examples of art that conveyed to them a sense of strength or weakness and to take photos for sharing later with their classmates.

The museum curator, Adera, talked about the Biederman piece for a few minutes, pointing out the shadows, the perspective changing depending on where a viewer might stand. Adera joked about Laurie being her lovely, taller assistant, who would demonstrate this looking exercise.

"What part of this looks strongest to you?"

Students spoke into the circle at random, sometime affirming or disagreeing with what others said: *The shadows. The pieces parallel to the ground. The blue canvas itself, like the blue of sky and earth.*

"See how the blocks are lining up like a ladder but don't overshadow the ones below?" said one student. "It reminds me of the way every person on a team might be at a different level but not be overshadowed."

"What part of this looks weakest?" Adera asked.

Students spoke again. *The smaller squares. The orange ones look ready to slide off. The isolated squares.*

"The strong and weak come together in this work of art to form one compositionally sound whole," Adera summarized. "This is true in life as well." She paused to let that sink in. We handed out paper that contained the journaling prompts as she read aloud.

"Think about a time in the clinical environment over the last few weeks when you've witnessed both strength and weakness in someone else. This person could be a patient, a family member, a fellow clinician, or even your supervising attending. Take a few minutes to write about that. Next, think about another recent clinical experience (it could be the same experience or another one) in which you've felt both strong and weak. Write about this."

We gave the students about thirty minutes to write in their journals on those two topics. Next the students moved into groups of twos and threes to share their reflections aloud. In small groups it is often easier to hear ourselves speak aloud for the first time what has gone unsaid, although it has been felt strongly in our hearts and heads. After small-group conversations, everyone rejoined the entire group and was invited to share, but only if they so chose. I always make sure to say it's never a "share or die" event and that remaining silent is just as valid. It's common for at least one student to choose to participate simply by listening rather than speaking.

That day, several medical students shared examples of patients who accepted their diagnosis with a strength of spirit. Other examples included physicians who showed confidence in their expertise but delivered news to their patients without empathy, which the students viewed as a weakness. More than one student told of seeing both strength and weakness in parents of sick children.

"A mother and father came to the ED with a ten-year old son who was autistic. The parents were so strong to have raised him so long but they no longer felt they could keep him safe. They felt they had to institutionalize him. They were strong people, and saints, but they were sobbing because they couldn't help their own son."

When we moved into the discussion about noticing their own strengths or weakness, the students gave examples of feeling weak for being unable to do more for their patients due to their inexperience. Many spoke of feeling frustrated at their own powerlessness against the human body's individual course of healing, about mental conditions that affected a patient's physical strength, and about the home life or personal conditions that influenced patient outcomes. That's when Mary shared her story.

## Time of Death

I had planned a three-hour session with the students that day but decided instead to spend more time exploring Mary's confession about feeling responsible for her patient's death and how she cried by herself in the stairwell. "Let's take a moment. I'm happy to share what I do when a patient I have cared for dies. I try to be mindful of my feelings and take my own time to acknowledge them."

I described to the group what I do and say to my team at times when a patient dies or we lose a patient to unsuccessful resuscitation. "Can we take a few moments to be quiet, to bow our heads and be silent and present in whatever way we are called to be." If we have cared for the patient and know the patient, we offer gratitude to the patient to honor their spirit. For example, I'll say, "We'd like to remember Miss Jones. Although I didn't get to know Miss Jones, she gave us the privilege in this hospital of helping us learn and letting us take care of her. Let's think of her as a healthy woman with a beautiful smile, perhaps a mother, a daughter, a wife." If we knew the patient, I might say "Remember when she told us about playing the piano, or picking up her grandchild. Let's think about that. Let's also have a moment of gratitude for ourselves to be given the privilege to care for patients."

It only takes two or three sacred minutes to stop for shared reflection around the time of death. It helps give meaning to the patient relationship, even if that relationship lasted only for a few minutes, hours, or a few days. It humanizes the relationship. It is another reminder to us that we are each spiritual beings in a human body.

We end every session at the Hunter Museum by collating the students' spoken and written reflections, summarized with anonymity. This response stands out to me, "This exercise let me see how I might cope with stresses of being a health provider. In this field we need to get better about dealing with these things when they happen, not later when we feel ready. I've learned that although it seems we don't have time to stop and process our emotions, it is in our best interest to do so."

## Humanizing Medicine with Intention

How do we humanize every encounter when we do not have the comfort and intentionality of the museum space, but when we must attend to a list of twenty patients, one after another? How does that list not become "patient 3038 with heart failure" or "patient 3041 with diabetes"?

I have a mindfulness practice I call "my doorknob sign." Before I knock and turn the doorknob to enter a patient's room, I take a split second to gather and remind myself, "I'm going to see Mr. Smith now, and he is the wonderful farmer who told me he won't give up chewing tobacco," or whatever happy information I remember. In this way I create an intention to connect with my patient despite my busyness.

Likewise, when I see a colleague coming down the hall, it's typical to say "How are you doing?" or respond simply with "Fine." Instead, I practice the intention to really see the other person, say hello, and not just walk away. By doing so, I am not only centering myself but giving myself and others an invitation to build a relationship.

Remaining calm and composed can be as simple as physical self-care, the most basic of Maslow's hierarchy of needs. I ask my learners, "Have you had lunch or breakfast? Do you want to go for coffee rounds?" Especially on long calls, I always carry a bag of assorted candy that I get from Costco or Sam's Club. That bag of candy is popular. I often say, "Hey guys, is it candy time?" One year I carried packets of saltine crackers in my pocket to have on hand for a student who didn't eat candy. I try to learn what each team member likes and bring that. Recent additions have been granola bars, Kind bars, jalapeño chips, and the extremely sour Warheads!

Meeting our physiological needs with snacks is one thing. Air, food, water, shelter, clothing and sleep are at the foundation of Maslow's hierarchy of needs. I also ask my learners,

"What is your happy place?" You might call our happy place the rung of safety and security on Maslow's ladder, or the next rung up of love and belonging. We talk about how to get there. Some people show a photo of their dog, or cat, or family. Some share a piece of music they listen to. Others may bring out a scripture verse or a quote they carry along. These are simple reminders to center ourselves, know that we need to do so, and remember that our happy place can be close to us.

I am known by my colleagues, residents, and students after challenging moments to say, "Okay, come on, let's have happy thoughts." When I was chair of medicine, I would sign my emails with "Happy Thoughts!" (I usually don't use emails to communicate or as conversations; I use emails to request conversations or face-to-face meetings.) One year the resident class gifted me with a red Littmann Classic III stethoscope engraved with the words "Happy Thoughts!" I still use it today, a decade later.

## Maslow's Needs and the Wellness Domains

These days when I give talks on physician well-being, I've begun combining Maslow's hierarchy of needs with the eight domains of wellness identified by the US Substance Abuse and Mental Health Administration (SAMSA).[2]

Well-being starts with self, which must be integrated into the environment where we live and work. We spend at least eight of our waking hours in the workplace. Physicians, nurses, or learners cannot be effective if we haven't met our basic needs and if we don't feel part of a community. We often stay in denial and make excuses to ourselves. But most systems, especially in this time of consumerism and commoditized health care, seem to only want workers who function from the top rung of self-actualization, those who are wise and who create quality outcomes. They forget that we must provide our community of workers with the basic fundamental needs. Program directors and education directors must ensure that our learners are well rested, that we've given them time and permission to get food and water, that they have a sense of physical security, that they belong to a community. Students may not have a local social support structure, so often we are their community. But if students feel we are only interested in them as commodities, it perpetuates the cycle of loneliness and feeling defeated. If you want to address well-being, start with the little things—which aren't so little, in fact. We owe this to ourselves as well.

For instance, when medical students and residents are assigned to long shifts in the emergency room, they feel isolated because they have to be there constantly and they don't have access to food "after hours" when the cafeteria is closed. Likewise, our students pointed out that they had no hooks in the bathroom to hang their white coats, which are so heavily laden with their diagnostic instruments—the stethoscope, the reflex hammer, a flashlight, and what we jokingly have named the "peripheral brains" such as a book on fast facts, an iPad, or smartphone. I encourage them to keep a granola bar or any other quick snack too. Things we carry in our coats change in volume over the years. Fresh interns have everything they might possibly need. At my stage, we might carry our patient notes and our stethoscopes and often our students hand us any other instruments we may need.

These issues came up the moment we got people in a room to voice their concerns and gave them the power, the voice and agency, and we assured them that their voices were important. Some issues were low-hanging fruit and easy to fix. We bought a staff refrigerator for the ER and we keep it stocked every day. We installed hooks in staff bathrooms.

Another issue that arose was security on our campus. It is a huge campus. It was brought to our attention that we do not have enough security patrolling overnight. Students walk from the library late at night to their cars parked in an open garage, and nurses leave at all hours of darkness. We are now working hard with the support of our well-being task force to get more security cameras and a larger security force.

Our learners are not the only ones who get tired, upset, angry, and burned out. The requirements for electronic health records (EHR) can be so frustrating. I hear this all the time from students, residents, and even faculty: "I have to get my notes done!" I tell them I sometimes feel like screaming that I can't take this EHR anymore. In fact, I am a technophobe, having being exposed to digital communications as an adult. When I shared that frustration and actually invited my younger colleagues and learners to help me, we could relate on a human level. I don't have to show I am an expert. I only show them that we are in this together and can find a solution.

I try to ease their minds. "I understand we have conflicting responsibilities. We can't align our mission around why such detailed documentation is mandatory when we just want to go take care of a patient and document only what's absolutely needed. We don't have a full understanding of why our national and local stakeholders want us to do this."

I empathize, try to reassure them that their voice is being heard and represented. It's more complicated than it looks, but we are working toward change. I try to empower them, "You are the boots on the ground. You are the ones utilizing the EHR more than we as faculty. We need your feedback."

Communication with each other within the hospital is equally frustrating. Physicians have to carry pagers and then we get direct calls on our cell phones from nurses. One resident told me, "I am carrying six pagers on my belt. I'm completely stressed and burned out."

We discussed this issue at the residency advisory board that I chair with resident representatives from all the different departments and leadership from the university and hospital.

Now we are working with our information technology department for a solution. They have assigned an individual who is a blackbelt in patient safety and quality improvement to work solely on this. Contributing valuable ideas and information helps our residents feel empowered now. Something that was frustrating is now a catalyst for changing the entire organization towards a culture of well-being. We are giving them a voice and empowering them to be part of the solution.

Some are relatively simple issues. We must look at well-being beyond yoga and mindfulness, which of course are important. Empowering people to speak up about their needs requires the psychological safety to speak without repercussion and to see evidence that their concerns will be listened to and solved together, and from that safety comes a sense belonging.

Belonging is vital. We have an epidemic of loneliness, which has been cited by a former US surgeon general as one of the top causes of burnout.[3] Health care has become a system based on shift work and no longer feels like one of camaraderie. I recently met with a group of seasoned physicians to talk about this. The conversation sounded like this: "In our day, we used to sit down and talk over a cup of coffee, or beer and pizza. We never do that anymore. Now we come in, looking at our iPhones or the computer screen. We have too many patients to see. We go home and complete our work there in our pajamas. We hardly see the colleagues we work with. We work so hard during our shift, then the next shift comes in and our paths never cross."

Community has been lost, in large part due to the hours spent instead on required electronic health records.[4] It's important to create opportunities for people to get together on a social basis—simply making the invitation matters. Making time for conversation matters.

## Recharging in Real Time

I precept on the inpatient wards for a short time every month. The team represents all levels of learners—residents, medical students, pharmacist, and physician-assistant (PA) students. To be able to work as a whole team requires keeping a pulse on the temperature of the team. I say we have to be thermostats, not thermometers. We have to be calm and composed ourselves because we are meeting our patients and families at their worst times.

I like to pick a time when we're not rushed, toward the end of the day when we're winding down. There are big windows on a few of the hospital floors where we can see the bridge over the Tennessee River—it's a beautiful view. I prefer to gather students in this spacious, sunlit lobby so that we can get recharged by looking out into nature. Our physical environment can be a barrier to physician well-being. In the winter, arriving and leaving the hospital in the dark can cause seasonal affective disorder.

I tell them, "You spend most of your time looking at your computers, let's pause for a bit."

The team sits back, discussing what loose ends need tied up, recapping the day. I pass the candy bag around the circle. Depending on the week, at the end of a rotation, I will say, "We've had a good time together and learned a lot. We had the opportunity to take care of patients."

Then I ask them to reflect on three questions. *What gave you hope? What inspired you? What surprised you?*"

We take time to think about those three questions. It's as useful to me as it is for the team. We discuss what helped us, what made us better, and how we were touched by our patients in a way that was unique to this experience?

Reflection often works best when you can contrast the positive with the more challenging or negative situations.

## A Tale of Two Patients

One week we cared for an 80-year-old gentleman from the countryside of rural Tennessee. He was in the end-stages of his cancer with a lot of pain and discomfort. Every day I'd go in, knowing we were trying to make him comfortable and prepare him for the end-of-life conversations. When I met him, he had already been in the hospital for more than ten days. He was tired and exhausted. With his nearly toothless smile, he was always quick with a joke. He greeted me by saying I was beautiful. We were able to laugh about our respective accents, which were both a little hard for the other to understand.

One day he asked aloud, "How do people find it in themselves to be strong?" It was the day before he was going to be discharged with hospice care, and his daughter was there too. He didn't seem to need an answer. He just looked at me and said, "You've been very kind. I will never forget you."

"Me neither," I said. "I will always remember your smile." His daughter and I were both crying. The team was behind me. I used to be ashamed of and hid my tears, but not anymore. I carry in my pocket small heart-shaped stones I call "healing hearts" and gave him one.

That evening at precept circle, this patient was mentioned many times.

One student said, "I feel so sad that I can't do anything for the patient." Another said, "I wish I had more time to sit and listen to his stories. I bet he had so many fun stories."

Only one resident actually took care of this patient (we divide patients among team), but this 80-year old man also touched those who didn't care for him directly. The residents saw that inspiration not only comes from the patient but the family. Hope comes from giving *care* not *cure*. We discussed how to remain positive despite knowing the end is in sight.

The same week we had quite the opposite situation. There

was a young man who did everything to jeopardize his own health. He was labeled as a difficult patient because he continued to make lifestyle choices that were detrimental to his health, such as IV drug use, smoking. He required heart surgery due to the damage from IV drug abuse.

The residents voiced complaints about this patient. "He's always wanting pain meds or wanting to go out for a smoke."

I was struck by the different emotions toward our two patients, both very sick but for one there was empathy and the other, frustration. One student noted the cliché question, "why do the worst things happen to the best people?" We often deal with this paradox—some patients we can relate to, others we cannot. How do we overcome our biases and see such a person as a human crying out for help? It's our job and duty, a tenet of our oath, to help irrespective of where the patient comes from.

Reflective questions are rarely resolved in a single conversation. If we create a safe space to talk with others about the soul-deep questions of our profession and our lives, we begin to understand that we have these feelings as humans and we can learn to hold the paradoxes. The goal of such conversations is not to find answers, nor to fix or save each other, but to give us permission to be human. Mindful reflection allows us to give voice to our emotions in a meaningful way. Simply hearing the shared thoughts of others helps us look in the mirror for ourselves. That is why reflecting (or being introspective) in a supportive community can nurture our resilience.

*What gave you hope? What inspired you? What surprised you?* By bringing the team together to find meaning in our work, the conversation reminds us to reconnect our passion to our purpose and recharge each day. I hope my learners ask themselves these questions every day, even if I'm not there. Making time to reclaim meaning in one's work is a vital form of self-care.

*Self-care is never a selfish act—it is simply good stewardship
of the only gift I have, the gift I was put on earth to offer
others. Anytime we can listen to true self, and give it the
care it requires, we do so not only for ourselves, but for
the many lives we touch.*

PARKER J. PALMER

## 18  TOUCHING OF THE FEET

*When we bless others, we offer them refuge from an*
*indifferent world.*

RACHEL NAOMI REMEN

I FEEL immense gratitude for my parents and kids. I always knew that my family was a blessing, but my dark times help me realize the magnitude of the blessing. After surviving my stress and sorrow, I wanted to give back.

When it came time to celebrate my parents' fiftieth wedding anniversary, I decided to honor them with a festive celebration in India, a surprise complete with extended family plus life-long friends who are part of our soul family. Family is important to my parents and both are the eldest sibling in their families. Despite my firm belief that "family is not blood," I wanted Natasha and Nik to feel the essence of their Indian relatives with a big family reunion. They had heard about my extended family, but were too young to remember meeting them before we moved to America. Besides, I love planning surprise parties.

It soon became overwhelming to coordinate ideal travel

dates for more than twenty people from around the globe. While their anniversary date is November 26th, only the last week of December was feasible for everyone. During college, Nik belonged to a fraternity with eleven other "brothers." They had all committed to spending every New Year's Eve together. Nik reminded me of this promise when I called to tell him the date of the anniversary trip and party.

"Can I bring a friend?" Nik asked, referring to his college roommate, valuing both family and friends.

"Yes, of course!"

Within a few hours, one guest for Nik became all eleven fraternity brothers. So now I was arranging a trip with twelve young men, my daughter and her two friends, myself and two of my close colleagues. The planning was becoming more than I could handle from America. Finally, I let my parents in on the secret so they could help. They happily arranged for guests to stay in nearby homes, while immediate family stayed at their home. About fifty relatives from India, including second and third cousins, would descend on Goa for a four-day event.

Finally, December came and I flew to India with Nik and most of his fraternity brothers. We connected with more of our party who met us at the Delhi airport for the final flight to Goa. Natasha met us there with a mini bus. My dad, mom, and my Aunty had prepared a large volume of delicious food, and they welcomed everyone warmly.

Natasha choreographed a tribute dance representing styles of Indian dance across the five decades to depict my parent's life. In each dance she included friends and family, youngest to oldest. She invited Nik's fraternity brothers to be part of the dance, and they all practiced in the living room, dancing away, Natasha with henna on her hands.

On December 29th, a traditional Indian prayer ceremony (puja) took place in the temple, complete with all the rituals and traditions. My parents retook their wedding vows. It was an emotional time. A reception followed at the hotel grounds. All that practice paid off when the dance was perfect and the boys received accolades at the reception (and again at a New Year's Eve party where they reenacted the dance just for fun).

Our Brahmin tradition in India is for the family and friends to touch the elders' feet for their blessings. We do this not only at weddings, but as a form of greeting and farewell, or at the beginning or completion of any auspicious event. Literally, you are supposed to touch the feet, but many people simply bow from their waist toward the feet of an elder as a sign of great respect. At the conclusion of the puja, many family and friends lined up to touch my parents' feet for their blessing, while others watched on the sideline. The air was solemn and heavy with emotion as each member touched my parents' feet, with only a few words quietly exchanged, sometimes only nods. Many families posed with my parents for a picture. Natasha, Nik, and I also had silently made our way from the end of the line. After Nik touched my parents' feet, and without any prompting, his friends from America also came forward and touched my parents' feet in reverence to receive their blessings.

When Nik was much younger, he was embarrassed to touch feet in public places. I would often say to him back then, "This is our way of showing respect. Don't be ashamed." As he matured he was proud to honor and share our culture spontaneously. For his friends to touch his grandparents' feet was such a silent yet significant ways of modeling what is meaningful to our culture. My dad had tears in his eyes because he already felt close to these boys. We were all so touched by their gesture and proud of Nik.

During that week in India for the anniversary party, my dad would enjoy a game of Carrom with Nik and his friends. When they left, my dad joined Facebook to stay in touch with them. He was delighted to learn a few years later that one of Nik's friends bought a Carrom game board to take to his Teach for America assignment.

The following May, Nik graduated from the University of Virginia, an occasion for my parents and our family to celebrate again. As soon as Nik's friends saw my parents, they went and touched their feet—in front of everyone. Several parents at graduation told me how their sons' friendship with Nik and traveling to India was such a life-changing cultural experience for their sons. My son made me proud, made us proud!

Years later at Nik's wedding, his friends all came, one boy noting Natasha was like their elder sister. As before, all the boys went to touch the grandparents' feet.

A person's home is blessed by the number of shoes outside the front door. During the anniversary party week, we had over one-hundred shoes outside my parent's door. Blessings indeed when we can weave our friends and family together in joy.

## An Unexpected Angel

Family is not blood. It's a truth I kept seeing. Making my way briskly down the hospital hall to see one of my residents' patients, I was stopped short by a phone call from my mother. My parents were in Saudi Arabia. My dad had just been taken to the hospital and was to undergo dialysis. He was in serious trouble. My heart lurched. In a flash, how life makes a complete about-face.

As I walked with more measured steps into the room where the patient was lying quietly, I saw that a member of the housekeeping staff was also there and the two men were praying. The custodian quickly apologized to me, gathered himself to exit, and reassured the patient that he would return later. It was obvious that daily prayer with this gentleman meant a great deal to our patient. I urged him to stay and continue praying, indicating that I would join them, "No, no. Don't leave. Prayer is important." In an attempt to validate my statement, I shared my belief, "We (physicians) are only instruments and we don't cure. We never give up hope."

As we stood praying by the patient's bed, tears sprang into my eyes. "Could you say a prayer for my dad?" The custodian asked where my father was specifically, and without missing a breath he continued to offer his intercessions.

I would encounter this kind man now and then as he unobtrusively went about his work at the hospital, and each time he would ask after my dad. For a space of two years, I missed seeing him, then one day there he was. He had lost weight, but his soft, clear eyes were unchanged. "I have been diagnosed with pancreatic cancer, but God will heal me. I have faith and I will be cured." And yes, once again he inquired sincerely about my family.

While I often spoke about him with my parents and prayed for him, it was nearly eighteen months later before I saw him again wearing his uniform working in the hospital corridors. I was so happy. It was wonderful to see him again. Though it had been quite a long time, our conversations were still powered by the grace and mercy of God. We voiced our shared gratitude and joy that he was back and healthy.

"The doctors told me I am cured," he told me, giving his God the glory. He and I both knew that often the prognosis with pancreatic cancer is palliative and not curative. After that, I would continue to see him on various occasions during my hospital rounds. We always acknowledged each other and, when time permitted, took a moment to inquire about each other and our families. Each time he assured me that he was continuing to pray for me and my family. I told him I too prayed for him and his family. Whenever I had an issue that was worrying me, or I was awaiting any important information, it seemed I would run into him. Though I did not share any of my concerns, his reassurance of prayer and need to trust God was relieving. My belief in confirmations strengthened!

Five years after first meeting him, my mother was ill. On my way to the procedure prep room, who did I see? It was my housekeeping/heart-keeping friend, appearing again in a time of need. By now he had added a term of endearment to our brief exchanges. "How are you, doll?" followed by, "And how is your dad?"

"Let me show you," I smiled back, thankful to see him, and took him to the room where my father waited. Naturally, we prayed together. After that, we began communicating via text. At random points throughout a day, up would pop a message such as, "Thinking about you." "Wow!" I would text in return, "Say a prayer for my mom." He asked that I call him to let him know how my mother was doing. Before I had a chance to call, he had sent another caring text message, "God is good." These confirmations of timely reassurances continue.

Always now, each morning, we have a virtual buddy check, exchanging thoughtful words in a text message. Whenever we see each other at work, my friend never passes by without a warm greeting, a little hug, and a "How is that sweet family of yours?" Then off we go on our separate ways.

This man of a humble heart is an angel in my life, one who delivers reassuring messages from the love of God. Every Diwali—the Hindu New Year and a celebration of the good over the evil—I have a traditional celebration at home. He is so happy to come and be part of a large family and friends celebration. He and my dad have good conversations.

Over the years, I have learned more about him, his love for music, his grandchildren, and that he is widowed and an usher in his church. Oh, and yes, his health has all the appearances of having stabilized.

·   ·   ·

FAMILY DOES NOT HAVE to be blood, as my daughter once said. I really believe that. Some angels come and go, some are in the background of one's life, and others stay with us out of gratitude or grace and keep on giving. I certainly have been blessed by many more than the few I have shared. Any time my family has needed a father or uncle figure, a friend or sister, someone would always come to fill that role. When we moved across continents to the United States, my paternal uncle and aunt fulfilled the roles of parents to me and of grandparents to my children. They continue these roles through their extension of ever present and unwavering support. Similarly, I know that I can call upon my younger brothers anytime.

I feel these connections now and so I am more receptive to them than I once was. There was once a time when I wanted to analyze these experiences to extract every particle of their fullness. Now, because I know that God sends insights through his grace, I instead pray for God's help to experience his gifts according to his will.

Living life often feels like we are forced to hold the tension between overthinking and anxiety-provoking brooding. This can be exhausting in every way. I grew up with parents and grandparents who were optimistic. My grandparents believed, role modeled, and drew solace from their optimism and faith. They accepted (and taught) that whatever happens is for your highest good and purpose. This concept is the basis of my belief in something bigger and more knowledgeable than myself who cares for my well-being.

Surrendering to this higher power reminds me that I am here to do what I can with the gifts I am given. Every human is given a purpose. Mine is to live for others. To do that is an unconditional surrender to the higher being. Therefore, I need to fulfill my role to my best ability with genuine effort and accept the outcomes.

Surrendering is hard. It evokes frustrations and impatience, anger and guilt, and all sorts of emotions. It is the journey of living, through prayer, kindness, and forgiveness for myself and others, including true honest feedback (even if harsh) from genuine friends and family, as well as inspiring role modeling from the same.

—

*I am blessed to have so many great things in my life—*
*family, friends and God. All will be in my thoughts daily.*

LIL' KIM

## 19  WHAT AM I FIGHTING FOR?

*There is in us an instinct for newness, for renewal, for a*
*liberation of creative power. We seek to awaken in*
*ourselves a force which really changes our lives*
*from within.*

THOMAS MERTON

"IF YOU WANT to see God laugh, tell him your plans!" I saw
these words on a billboard in front of a church over a decade
ago, during my daily commute to and from work. I smiled then,
yet felt a solemn realization of the need for unconditional
surrender.

Life happens! I am a strong believer that our lives move in
cycles just like the seasons. Seasons have the power to shape
our feelings, attributes, and behavior. Every time of year, it
seems, brings its own formative influences. I thought I had
been mindful in preparing to live through each season of my
life with faith and trust. However, actually living through a dark
season is a different realization.

It was July of 2017 when my back began to ache after a trip

to Japan. I had given a presentation in Osaka and then spent a few extra days vacationing with my friend Indrani. I saw an orthopedic surgeon, who ordered an X-ray and an MRI. Those showed slight evidence of a disc problem. I asked the orthopedic surgeon, "Do you think I can travel?" I had already scheduled in late August to fly to India with Nik and his fiancé, Anuja, and her parents. We were going to meet and celebrate with her family who would be unable to attend the wedding in America the following summer. And we planned to shop for the traditional festive Indian clothes for the bride, groom, parents, and the bridal party, and some traditional decorations too.

The surgeon said "Yes, do your prescribed physical therapy, let your body be your guide, and you will be better and able to travel." He gave me a tapering steroid dose pack. By mid-August I felt good enough to take the trip to India as planned.

I was very careful about what shoes I wore, where I walked, and doing my stretches. We had rented an Airbnb apartment and were all staying there together. The day we were leaving to come home from India, there was torrential, tornado-type rain in Mumbai. Our flight was not until evening, leaving us time to do some final shopping.

But early that morning, Anuja's dad woke us, saying, "Look, we're going to pack, vacate the house, and go now. We will do what we can on the way to the airport because soon we will not be able to drive in this rain." We looked at him with dismay. He could see on our faces that we were questioning his logic without saying aloud what we were each thinking. *What? Our flight is not until seven o'clock. That's twelve hours from now.*

He replied to our unspoken words, "I know the monsoons in India. Let us get out as soon as possible." Well, we didn't want to argue with him, so we quickly rushed and packed. We were definitely not prepared for this sudden ending. And I think we were a little disappointed because Anuja and Nik had an appointment to try on their wedding clothes and be measured for alterations and we had some decorations to buy. But her dad was so right! By the time we left the apartment, the rain was coming down hard. The umbrellas did not protect us from becoming soaked as we raced to the car with our suitcases. Water was already collecting on the streets. We had just enough time to get to the clothing store for Anuja and Nik to have their fitting. They frantically and prayerfully asked for reassurance to continue the alteration conversations via email and Facetime. As we left the store about forty-five minutes later, we were driving in water three and four feet deep. Anuja's dad, Anuja, and Natasha ended up making another trip six months later to continue the special shopping we couldn't finish that day.

How Anuja's dad drove us to the airport that day is miraculous. The typical hour-long journey took closer to two and half. He really deserves credit not just for his driving skills, but for remaining calm, focused, reassuring, and positive. But the potholes! He couldn't see them underwater and couldn't avoid them if he wanted to! I was in the backseat with Anuja and her mom, and we were just being thrown up and down, up and down, up and down. That's when my back started hurting more. When I got to the airport, I took a couple of Aleve. I was really praying for my back. *I hope everything's okay.*

We had a seven-hour wait until our flights. Luckily, customs were not busy. I had a pass to the airline lounge. The attendant took pity on us, tired and drenched, and allowed me to bring Anuja and Nik into the lounge too. Before we checked in our luggage, we had the presence to remove a change of clothes for each of us. It felt good to put on dry clothes and have a warm meal. My flight was not delayed, but Anuja and Nik were traveling to Boston on another flight thirty minutes after mine. Theirs was delayed a few hours.

During my seventeen-hour flight to Atlanta I could feel the

backache worsening. I took Tylenol and Aleve throughout the flight, and even had two glasses of wine despite knowing full well I really shouldn't. The customs line was longer in Atlanta than Mumbai. After another hour wait, I boarded the final flight to Chattanooga, my pain increasing, my body longing for a hot bath and my bed. I arrived home about twenty-two hours after leaving Mumbai.

The next day I had some tingling and numbness in my left leg, and it wasn't going away. That's when I got really scared and upset. After four days I went back to see the orthopedic surgeon again and he said, "You definitely have a disc hernia-tion. And it's going to take time to get better."

## Suddenly in a Patient's Shoes

In that split second of a confirmed diagnosis, my role changed from that of a physician to patient. Although it had been building over several months—with my back-to-back overseas travels, the trauma of bouncing over monsoon potholes, sitting on planes—it was that moment when my predicament became real.

The pain became so severe, it was unbearable. I couldn't lift anything heavy, not even a gallon of milk into the fridge. I couldn't load and unload the dishwasher. I couldn't bend down to put my laundry in the washer and dryer. Getting up the stairs was painful. I was thinking, "I'm all alone. Who is going to take care of me?" My parents delayed going back to India to stay and care for me. (They usually spend about three months in India and nine months in America mostly with me and some with my brother in New Jersey.)

I was paralyzed in pain and feared I would never walk again. I couldn't wear heels. I could only wear flat shoes. You know, this thought crossed my mind, *What if I could never again wear cute shoes with heels?* And physical therapy just made the pain worse.

The next day I went to the department chair to discuss my diagnosis and my options. Getting in and out of the car was painful. I walked slowly in obvious pain, wearing my comfortable tennis shoes. "I can't walk very far," I told him. "I can't do inpatient teaching and calls."

"Well, I support you taking the time you need," he said, "but I would prefer you apply for the Family Medical Leave Act. You have enough leave, so that way nobody can question your time off."

Another issue was weighing heavily on my mind. This was the time of year when I had to write the medical student performance evaluations for the students in their final year, to accompany their electronic application to residency programs. I was the only one responsible for this task for the students at the Chattanooga campus. While it was simply desk work, people might think I was getting preferential treatment if I came just to do some things and not do other things. The thought of that hurt, but I understood. I agreed to apply for medical leave and to stay home.

After getting the department chair's approval for leave, I went to the dean's office. He also said, "Absolutely." I was grateful for the university's staff help to complete the FMLA paper work that same afternoon. I was reminded of how complicated and convoluted navigating such processes are. While I knew people who could speak for me and help, what about those who have no one who can be their voice?

I did work from home to meet the obligations to the six students who still needed their letters completed. Life happens suddenly, but we have commitments. These students who needed recommendations letters would have suffered if I hadn't written their letters, and it would have been difficult for me to live with those consequences. True, the students could have travelled five hours by car to Memphis where other faculty could have completed these letters. But I did not want to inconvenience them and add to their already stressful time. Some came to my home where I did their interviews and wrote their letters.

One lesson I learned from this situation is to make sure I'm not the only person capable of writing recommendation letters. Cross-training is important.

I must admit, I did do other work from home. Physicians rarely give ourselves the time to heal, but it's difficult to define where the boundary is between self-care and our responsibility to others. (Of course, this problem isn't limited to physicians.) If you view the FMLA rules only by the book, you wouldn't work at all. I justified it in my mind, *I'm doing this on my own time.* We do so as human beings, not just physicians, because to do so aligns with our moral compass.

It would be nice to be in a community of people who would create a system around us so that we do not find ourselves in this position, where we've done the cross training, and we feel permission to say "I can't do this, can you help me?" I have to take ownership to help build a different system, and to build a community going forward, because I'm not the only one in this situation.

## Despair and Depression

That September and October of medical leave were very hard. I am grateful my parents were there to care for me, and simply as loving parents, not wearing their physician hats. They would comfort me when I would cry from the pain of the muscle spasms. The pain wasn't going away. What else could be happening? I dreamt that I had other causes of back pain, like ovarian cancer or colon cancer. All of these bad thoughts were going through my mind.

I became depressed, mainly from a feeling of dependence. I didn't want to be a burden on my parents or, long-term, on my kids. Also, I was so scared that I couldn't do what I had planned. I had to cancel a trip to Dharamshala, the Dalai Lama's place of residence, and a trip with Indrani to the Golden Temple and the India/Pakistan border. I had to cancel a lecture at a conference. I couldn't do all the things that were normally routine. It may sound so trivial, but I really couldn't wear my fun shoes! That was depressing, too!

I found myself going through all the stages of denial, anger, bargaining, depression, and acceptance. But then, after a couple of weeks of wallowing in my own pity party, my faith and convictions cleared my thinking. My faith and prayer gave me strength.

I started asking myself questions: *What do I really want? Suppose something like this really is happening? What if I never get back to 100% so that I can travel or wear heels again or be out of pain completely? What if I can never go back to my "normal" life as if this obstacle had never happened? If that is the case, then what is it that am I fighting for?*

You know, I told myself, institutions and recognitions are not going to give me comfort and joy. My relationships and my family and friends are. The community that I have. And what can I do to really celebrate that fact, affirm that, cultivate that? But more importantly, what can I do to really *contribute* to that?

Exploring that line of thought became so important. It helped me create a different mindset of inner healing to support my physical recovery.

## More Than Physical Healing

I can't do sitting meditation. To me, walking is meditation. My routine is to walk in silence for three to five miles. I walk at a very brisk pace listening to music, my spiritual, pop, or Bollywood songs, depending on my mood. I'm listening but not listening, ruminating on things in my mind. Sometimes I walk with a colleague. If I don't walk, I feel like I missed out.

With my herniated disc, the normalcy of my life was taken away. Since I couldn't walk, I focused on a breathing meditation. I visualized the chakras (the balls of energy) in my body. I visualized my breath as a white light going through the chakras and coming out. Centering myself and focusing with meditation helped me get my inner strength back.

This was a period of time when I wanted to hold onto anything people told me would help. A dear friend, who also had a herniated disc the year before, and her sister put me in touch with YouTube meditation videos and techniques for healing. The videos were helpful because I am a visual person. It got me focused on something different.

Walking the path as a patient calls upon mustering every ounce of faith and courage you possess and holding onto the constant thread that sustains you through an ever-changing life. It was no different for me.

The journey was hard, through terrain I had never treaded. I was not equipped with the right gear. I questioned whether I should have pursued physical yoga more earnestly. It did not interest me on the few occasions I tried, but would that have helped me heal faster? I felt guilty that I questioned my faith initially. *Had I failed to prepare adequately? Could I have prepared adequately?*

Physical healing took almost a year, although even now, years later, I am still not one-hundred percent pain free. I still continue physical therapy. My attitude toward this pain is one of acceptance. I'm doing better day by day.

The mental healing was quicker than the physical healing. This depression was short-lived and situational. Other incidents in life ten years earlier had prepared me for that time. We don't always understand the gift we have in our challenges because we only have hindsight. That's why sometimes you just have to trust—and maybe that's where surrender comes in.

This back pain made me understand who I reach for when I'm desperate. It solidified for me my faith, but also that my faith is active. For me, daily living is a prayer and having faith is not just a belief. I have to do something to make sure that faith continues, whether it's though meditation, reading, or prayer. Or leaning on friends and family for support.

## Fighting for Joy and Belonging

I began my "relationship board" in 1998 when I became faculty. It is a cork bulletin board measuring about four by four feet in size. It started in July when I received a photo from one of my colleagues who had a new baby that I loved to hold. (I have been known as baby whisperer.) I would always ask his wife to bring the baby for my "baby therapy." And then I added photos of the new students and others. In December that year I started getting Christmas cards from my residents, many with photos of them with their spouses and children. Then wedding invitations came. The board was such a great conversation starter. The nurses would stop by my office and say things like "Oh, I remember this guy." When I became department chair and moved to a bigger office, I requested an even bigger board. I said, "I need this." That's when I started adding positive quotes. More pictures grew in over the quotes, which were over earlier pictures. And now I have more than two decades of pictures over pictures over pictures. I finally added a smaller board beneath it.

To me, this relationship board represents the difference between joy and happiness. Joy is not a choice. Joy is something you have to choose to cultivate. I read that somewhere. I can't take full credit for it, but I have to expand on it a little bit. To me, joy is very much a "relationship emotion." Joy is a deeper

Namaste. *I not only see this worth in your spirit and welcome it, but I can feel a connection between us as human beings.*

Happiness is one of the manifestations of joy. But it doesn't need to be relationship oriented. Happiness can be fleeting or superficial. I'm happy when I get a good piece of chocolate. I am happy when I see the rain after a warm day. But when I'm anticipating a meaningful conversation, that brings me joy. When I'm in conversation and it's evoking different emotions, this is joy, and I want to experience more of it. Happiness can be trivial, but joy wants me to go back to the experience. Joy is addictive. Once I cultivate that joy both with passion and compassion, then I have that relationship. It's a relationship with joy as well as a relationship with another person.

Whether the other person reciprocates or not, you can appreciate your own feeling of being present authentically. I can choose to connect with others in joy irrespective of whether the relationship is reciprocated. Making the attempt feels gratifying. There's only so much I can do to build a relationship. I've done something I could do—and that's all that is in my power. Sometimes I want to protect myself from harm. I may go out of my way to be kind, but get a rebuttal. I learn through experience, through successes and failures. By unpacking what happened, I see what I need to fill my own soul so that I have more joy to give to others.

An emotional, visceral feeling comes over me when I look at my relationship board. My door is never closed. I don't lock my door. One day a staff person was in my office as we were trying to navigate through bylaws and requirements that were being implemented soon. It so happened that she was really frustrated at the care that a family member was receiving and needed to vent about it. She sat down facing the board. After a few minutes, she said, "It just gives me such peace looking at this."

My relationship board is not a decorative wall-hanging. It

represents my sense of belonging to a community of caring, loving, compassionate people. When I think of my years-long question, "How do I heal as I strive to serve?" the answer that comes to mind is one word: *Belonging.* I used to think my other guiding question was "Where do I belong?" As I lived into the question longer, I began wondering if I was really asking, "*How do I belong?*" My answer to how—how to belong, how to heal, how to serve—is through the joy and action of cultivating a community of belonging. I belong to a community which includes not only my friends and family, my colleagues, coworkers and learners, but my patients and their families.

## Fighting Against Destructive Altruism

On my journey through depression while healing from a herniated disc, I found myself asking the following questions:

*What am I fighting for? What is the fine line between productive passion and destructive passion? Is my self-perceived altruism pathologic? What is my purpose now? Where do I truly belong, not just pretend to blend in or fit in?*

These questions brought to mind the Thomas Merton quote about the violence of modern life:

> *To allow oneself to be carried away by a multitude of*
> *conflicting concerns, to surrender to too many demands,*
> *to commit oneself to too many projects, to want to help*
> *everyone in everything is to succumb to violence. The*
> *frenzy of the activist neutralizes his work for peace. It*
> *destroys the fruitfulness of her own work, because it kills*
> *the root of inner wisdom which makes work fruitful.*

It's so true. Our frenzy destroys the fruitfulness of our work. It's not just that many physicians inherently have a type-A competitive nature. But the system incentivizes and rewards such behavior. We have all perpetuated the system to a crisis point where we feel we must be workaholic multitasking superhumans.

Do we continue our frenzy under the guise of altruism? Is our passion coming from an altruism that is actually harmful and destructive to us? Who will give us permission to change the system? How do we begin to crack the layers of the conditions that developed over time? Change must come from different sources, including self.

Burnout amongst health care professionals, especially physicians, has reached epidemic proportions. Is it possible that our basic value of altruism is causing harm to ourselves and those we aim to help? The concept of pathological altruism is given thorough coverage in *Pathological Altruism*, an insightful book of academic papers edited by Barbara Oakley and team.[1] With so many people exploring this emerging field, we may come to better understand the unanticipated hurtful effects of altruism and empathy.

I invite reflection on more questions: Do I have to be altruistic in quantity, and when will that quantity be enough? Who decides that quantity? Have we used altruism as an excuse to drown our other issues, like not wanting to deal with our personal, professional, or family lives? Does altruism give us a driving force that gives us value—or is that value superficial?

How do we as health care professionals create an environment in which we honor our own experience and not lose sight of the core values that initially brought us to medicine and to leadership? How do we discern the fine line between restorative or replenishing altruism and what might actually be pathologic or destructive altruism?

Destructive passion may be another word for pathologic altruism. Destructive passion is destructive to self but also to family, to friends. When it leads to physician burnout, it is also destructive to the patient because burnout leads to an increase in physician errors and a decreased fulfillment and satisfaction with work. Passion is my strength, but it leads to my downfall when I pursue something to such a degree that I can't get the results I strive for. High expectations for myself drive overwork. That's where self-kindness and self-compassion come in. I wonder if destructive passion and pathologic altruism are not synonymous but related.

I don't have the answers. Institutions will not give me the answers. I remember the Russian folk story that asks how much land a man needs. The answer is that six feet of land is all you need at the end of the day, as in space for your coffin. Is it me growing old and cynical to think of this now? Am I being hypocritical to advise young physicians, "You really don't need to make these things a priority," meaning salary, accomplishment, recognition. I feel they are looking at me as if to say, "You're a fine one to say this now that you've achieved them." Or is it my duty, having understood some deeper meaning, to begin to hold the conversations about what gives life meaning?

## A Journey to Gratitude

I am grateful that my journey so far opened a door to these important questions, offering me a portal to explore myself over and over again. This journey taught me a level of compassion and empathy that was deeper and more personal. This journey reminded me again of the immense healing power of gratitude.

I can now truly say thank you for the gift of my back injury. It reminded me of the vital need for me to give myself permission for "Me time." That means taking time to acknowledge my emotions, not as right or wrong but with acceptance. Before, I would create stress by trying to justify or make excuses for my emotions, or come up with an answer to why. I am now more willing to tell myself, "This is how I'm feeling and I just have to be okay with it. I may understand why later." "Me time" also means making sure to take care of my physiological needs, and then finding family and community where I feel I'm safe and belong.

The experience of slow healing from my back pain gave more meaning to my fight to deliver medical care that includes mind-body-soul, not only the physical care of a person. It inspires me to fight for holistic health care even more. My fight is also a form of leadership to advocate for more intentional permission around physician self-care.

*Life is a C between B and D: Choices, Challenges and Confirmations between Birth and Death.*

MUKTA PANDA

# 20  MATCH DAY

*I WILL ATTEND TO my own health, well-being, and*
*abilities in order to provide care of the highest standard.*

THE DECLARATION OF GENEVA, REVISED 2017

MY LIFE as a teacher of medical students means that I cycle through the seasons with them. From September to February, I walk with them on their journey as they submit applications and interview for placement into their residency training program located in US teaching hospitals. During this season, fourth-year medical students in the US go on interviews, the majority done in person. Students compile their own rank list of the top places they'd like to go, noting how the possibilities match up to their hopes to be near home or another support system, near resources for pursuing their other passions and opportunities, or to have a certain education focus.

In 2017 I wrote those recommendation letters from home as I was struggling to recover from my herniated disc. Rather than walking with my students on rounds in the hospital that autumn, where I often heard about their residency interviews, I was on medical leave. Instead I would check in with them by email, or in conversations at my home or on the phone.

Every February I schedule a special session at the Hunter Museum of American Art. We revisit the Hippocratic Oath and explore its relevance and applicability to the current health care environment. I ask my senior graduating medical students to rewrite their own version of the Hippocratic Oath. In the museum's art studio, they can write their oath, draw their oath, or create their oath with materials of art. They read theirs aloud and we talk as a group. *How will you value the oath? What will happen if you don't? How will you deal with unexpected outcomes?* This exercise is part of their capstone course, which is required before moving on into residency training.

Every US and non-US medical student applies to residency at the same time with a common process. It's a big deal. The National Resident Matching Program is the single computerized system (which received an economic Nobel prize for its design[1]) that simultaneously matches more than 43,000 US and non-US applicants with 31,000 positions! As the director of my program, I interviewed approximately sixty student applicants and placed twenty or thirty of them on a rank list. These are my top choices—one, two, three—but I'll be happy with any of the others. The students do the same thing, ranking where they most want to go of all the places they interviewed. I encourage them to consider which place has resources, a support system, and which places are going to give them the education they desire. As efficient as it is, not every student is fully satisfied—and that's just the way it is.

Typically, on the Monday of the third week in March, students find out if they matched, but not until Friday at 1 p.m. Eastern time (and whatever is the corresponding time across the globe) do all students receive their envelopes. In the envelope is a sheet of paper that says, "Congratulations! You have matched at ...." Now, on that Monday, some students find out they haven't matched. Those students have until Thursday that week to go through what we call the "SOAP" or supplemental interviews where they can interview with programs that still have open slots. So in between Monday and Thursday, we help them secure a spot wherever they can.

That week is a very, very tense period of time for all of us. If any of our students don't get in elsewhere, our school has committed to give them a one-year placement.

On Friday we celebrate. The students come. Their families come. There's a wonderful meal, and Mimosas and Bloody Marys. And a ritual we co-create.

Each year as assistant dean of medical student education, I have asked the students "How would you like to receive your envelopes?" The first year, we put the envelopes on a table at the banquet hall at the Chattanoogan Hotel. The second year, I said, "Let's spice it up a little bit." My students asked to celebrate at the Hunter Museum of American Art, a space they treasured for all the afternoons there where we reflected on our well-being, meaning, and purpose. That year the students hung their envelopes on the walls the same way pictures are found in the galleries. With their envelope was their official graduation headshot and a photo of them as babies.

## Sudden Death

A medical student in Memphis had died by suicide just weeks before Match Day. He was someone my students knew from their first two years. News of his death traveled to East Tennessee fast. I found out about thirty minutes after my students. I felt immense sadness and anger. Sadness at the loss —no matter how, what, when, or why. My thoughts went to the many conversations with top leaders about prioritizing physician well-being, and I saw myself in the room yet again, *What data do we need to say it's too much? Now will you listen?* I was surprised by my attitude. *Do I need to have a tragic imperative every time? Am I trying to use this for leverage?*

I needed to be there for my Chattanooga students, right then and there. *How do I communicate and hold things together?* First, it was important to get the facts straight. I called the leadership in Memphis for details. Then one of my fourth-year medical students named Scott Ward called me. He was crying, telling me about the loss of his good friend. "Scott, where are you?" I asked, concerned for his safety. I know survivor's guilt can be heart-wrenching when you feel you could have and should have done more.

"I'm driving to Sewannee. I'm going to meet a friend."

"I want you to call me as soon as you reach there. Then call me tomorrow."

In the meantime, I convened a group of students. I invited the chaplain faculty because they have a very calming attitude. I sent out an email asking for grief resources to my Center for Courage & Renewal colleagues. In return, I soon received the poem "On the Death of the Beloved" by John O'Donohue and shared it with my students and colleagues when we gathered that day.

After that I would stay in touch with my students even more closely. I would offer, "Let's go for a cup of tea." Or they came to my office, my door always open. Two days before Match Day, Scott texted me a poem. At first, I didn't realize he was the poet.

*Fall is surely the best season.*
*The first leaf bronzes gracefully in its age, spreading its*
    *orange fire to its contemporaries, the veins of its life*
    *revealed by the sun.*
*Plucked by the wind, it embarks on its journey.*
*Independent at last, dancing joyfully on the autumn breeze.*
*Our friend is a harbinger of the color and life to come.*

*YET, in our rapture, let us not forget the sorrow of our leaf.*
*The pain that accompanies its loneliness.*
*The terror it faces in its fight with the wind.*
*The peace it embraces once resting on the ground.*

Scott asked if I would read it at the Match Day ceremony. The next day we talked a little more. I said, "I think you should read it."

"No, I don't think I can."

Instead we framed Scott's poem and placed it at Match Day with his friend's photo and an empty envelope as a tribute. Scott later read the poem in Memphis at his friend's memorial service. A year later in March, Scott sent me an email about the anniversary of his friend's death, saying, "Hey Dr. Panda. Thank you for all you did last spring. You made it a safe place to be."

In response to this student's suicide, university leadership worked with students to start an intervention program known as Campus CARES (Campus Awareness, Resources and Education).[2] This multidisciplinary team approach, which is available for all students at the four University of Tennessee campuses, provides a confidential way to identify students in or heading into distress, or with behavioral issues, so that they can get emotional, social, or academic support.

The following October 2018, another medical student at our Memphis campus died unexpectedly. The tragedy was another opportunity to talk with my students and colleagues about self-care and feelings of vulnerability. I am grateful for the established Hunter Museum sessions so our conversations could naturally focus for several months on the emotions of loss.

Together, these lost lives prompted a wellness initiative for the College of Medicine, which included updating policies that allow medical students to take time for physical and mental care, without question. Traditionally, medical students are often seen as being at the bottom of the totem pole and are not given standard time off for family and life obligations such as attending funerals or weddings, observing holy days, not even for maintaining their own health with preventative or elective health care appointments. A new wellness policy now helps our medical students establish a well-balanced lifestyle early in their medical careers.

## An Oath for Self-Care

In 2019 I again asked my students how they wanted to celebrate their Match Day. One student came up with a brilliant idea—piñatas! Students chose their own piñatas and we put their envelopes inside with candy. Students could bring the tool of their choice for breaking the piñatas open. We saw lacrosse sticks, broom sticks, baseball bats! Each piñata was hung on an IV pole (on wheels!), which their family held steady. The students had fun hitting the piñatas. Some screamed and cried joyfully. There was also a large map on a poster board. After reading their letter, each student walked up and placed their photo on the map wherever they were going for their residency.

The last moment of our Match Day celebration is to join in a circle, a tradition we established in our three years together. Looking around the circle you would see a dozen young men and women in casual business clothes, a feeling of anticipation and excitement, many smiles, some tears. A student who didn't get his number-one spot appeared upset.

"On your tables is a copy of the Declaration of Geneva," I said to the students, explaining the significance to their parents and grandparents. "This oath is known as the Modern-Day Physician's Pledge." I didn't tell them that the same October I was on medical leave for my herniated disc, the World Medical Association (WMA) General Assembly was meeting in Chicago where it adopted the recommendations of a working group to amend the Declaration of Geneva.[3] I didn't go into detail describing how the Declaration of Geneva was first written and adopted in 1947 to address the human and medical atrocities committed in World War II. I simply explained that it was written as an alternative code of ethics because the 2,500-year-old Oath of Hippocrates doesn't fully represent the challenges of the present. In 2017 new clauses were adopted, including a physician's commitment to self-care.

"We have spoken many times about our own self-care," I said, seeing the nods of my students, smiles exchanged among themselves. Perhaps they were recalling me talk about my own burnout, how I recognize my symptoms of sweaty palms, tension in the back of my neck, needing to take a brisk walk or to think of something positive, happy, or even imagining getting my anger out on a boxing bag until I can process my emotions later. On Match Day I challenged them (with reflective questions, of course) to stay aware of their well-being: "How do we make self-care an intentional part of our commitment to ourselves, our colleagues, and our vocation, and not something we just speak about? How do we intentionally work on making it a tenet we follow?"

"Students, please come up here into a circle. Let us all take the oath together."

The air in the room was quite solemn when they read the Declaration of Geneva aloud. As they read it, my eyes filled with tears. These students are truly part of the effort to institute a commitment to physician well-being. They've been so receptive and involved in well-being activities, particularly after the unexpected losses of two fellow med students.

After our time together, these students have developed strong roots and now wings to fly. They can continue this well-being work elsewhere and do even better work. I felt cheer, pride, and sadness, just as I did when my own children graduated and when each class of students moves on.

After reading the oath, we put our arms around each other

and stood in silence for another group hug. Their families laughed and applauded. Some had tears too.

## Empowered by Curiosity

While passion, being creative, and thinking outside the box are innate gifts I can claim with humble confidence as my strengths, they are also my weakness. Earlier in my life and career, I forged ahead without mindful reflection about how it was impacting me and the pulse of the audience around me, or the other members on the journey with me. But more recently I have learned that my impatience and frustration at my workplace was something I could control. I have learned to be gentle and allow my thoughts to be.

This is something that has been resonating with me more emphatically in the past few years, especially through intentionally reflecting and making myself go into the dark corners and shadows that are often easier to cover up, ignore, or deny.

The same has been true in my work of creating a culture of well-being, where we focus on being human—not just the best physician, student, or resident, but valuing each other as team members and human beings. While the topics of physical well-being, resiliency, and burnout are such buzzwords, I don't want them to be empty, meaningless words. I have to be mindful of approaching myself kindly as I navigate the cultural and political environment. I strive to build a culture of well-being, and that means being intentionally reflective, kind to myself and team members. That mindset has served me well.

However, in spite of that, part of me still gets upset. National political leaders must recognize the epidemic of physician burnout that has been identified by medical accrediting organizations and the former surgeon general Dr. Vivek Murthy. It must be put right up there with the opioid crisis. If this physician burnout epidemic were an infectious disease plaguing fifty to sixty percent of health professionals, or a serious cardiac disease crisis, the Centers for Disease Control (CDC) or the American Heart Association would put together a task force of like-minded intellectuals and experts, mandating a solution backed up with personnel and financial resources.

Oftentimes it feels like well-being is addressed as another item on the checklist of indicators required by the accrediting organization, like infection control in the hospital, or board passage rate of a training program. But burnout is different. This epidemic cannot and should not be addressed with a simple checkbox but must be addressed with a blending of both the mind and the heart. The difficulty often arises in the task of measurement. It takes intentionality, time, resources, and experience to quantify team engagement, physician empathy for patients, the meaning and purpose of work each day, all which contribute to a culture of well-being! For instance, the patient/physician relationship is a language of the heart, not a data point.

On one hand, it can be so frustrating and aggravating. On the other hand, I turn to a practice I was taught when I became a Center for Courage & Renewal Circle of Trust® facilitator, "When the going gets rough turn to wonder." I ask myself, *How can I turn to curiosity and discover what else can be done about this? I wonder what can we do to make this a community that cares?* That mindset is becoming easier because I have claimed the intention to be curious and interested rather than frustrated.

Many people in organizations have the right intention. I see myself continuing to build a community. When I engage with various stakeholders in workshops on physician resilience, I ask them to reflect on their personal statement to medical school or their residency application and remember what drew them to this profession in the first place. Almost unanimously they describe a connection of human relationship, whether this profession was a calling that came from having role models, or they built a relationship on a mission trip. We take time to reflect: *Where are you still connecting to your original passion and drive? What are the barriers to it? How can we reclaim that passion?*

Deep in our hearts we all seem to have a shared sense of why we're in this serving vocation. *How do we reconnect to our passion, purpose, and meaning?* I want to create safe and brave spaces where people can trust that if they speak openly about this personal connection, it will be celebrated and valued, not ridiculed as touchy-feely. That is how I've resolved to navigate this political environment. This is what I am fighting for.

*Every great dream begins with a dreamer. Always remember, you have within you the strength, the patience, and the passion to reach for the stars to change the world.*

HARRIET TUBMAN

## 21  RESILIENT THREADS

*I wanted a perfect ending. Now I've learned, the hard way,*
*that some poems don't rhyme, and some stories don't*
*have a clear beginning, middle, and end. Life is about not*
*knowing, having to change, taking the moment and*
*making the best of it, without knowing what's going to*
*happen next. Delicious Ambiguity.*

GILDA RADNER

"THE FIRST STITCH needs to be decisive, efficient, and quick! Everything depends on this first stitch!" The senior faculty advisor spoke these words during my first residency training in obstetrics and gynecology (OBGYN). Threads used to stitch can be life-saving, both literally and figuratively. This was even more apparent to me during my OBGYN training.

Our young patient had spent almost five months of her precious pregnancy laying in her bed at the hospital. She needed to be on complete bed rest until delivery, and both she and her unborn baby needed close monitoring. Thanks to the availability of high-quality ultrasound and regular antenatal care, she had been diagnosed with placenta previa. The placenta is the structure that provides oxygen and nutrients to the growing baby and removes waste products from the baby's blood. The condition in which the placenta partially or totally covers the mother's outlet from the uterus is known as placenta previa. This condition can cause severe bleeding throughout pregnancy and during delivery.

The team had come to know our patient and her husband well. We often saw her reading or doing crosswords puzzles. Our daily visits had taken on a mainly social flavor. Our questions were the same, so much so that she was ready with her answers even before we asked the questions, "The nurse told me my vitals are stable, my baby's heart rate is good, it is kicking like a football player. And I have no bleeding." We all were reassured!

However, this routine changed one eventful, busy morning. She had just reached thirty-two weeks of gestation and we all had spoken about how we had only a few more weeks to go until she could have an elective cesarean section to deliver the baby, who would be mature by then, with the least complications to baby and mother. We all prayed and hoped we would reach that time without complications.

Our team was on rounds when a nurse's loud scream interrupted our conversation. "I need help! My patient is bleeding!" We rushed in her direction, fearing the worst. We found a bloody scene. Our patient with placenta previa lay in a pool of blood, screaming in panic "Help me! Please, save my baby!"

The team sprang into action. With what felt like organized chaos, she was transferred to the operating room for an emergency caesarean section, the only way to save the baby and mother. This needed to be done quickly. Time mattered!

I was amazed. Our patient was rapidly being transfused with blood, but she was losing it faster than we could replace it.

I do not have a lot of details. I was the trainee and in the second assistant role.

It seemed surreal—and yes, a miracle—for in a few minutes I heard the baby cry as he was handed to the neonatal ICU staff who had been informed and were ready and waiting. Although few words were exchanged between the senior consultant, the head nurse, and my senior resident, as a team they communicated seamlessly.

I looked on, scared and praying. I was not sure how to be useful. I was not sure they knew I was in the room. My doubts were removed when the consultant's voice interrupted my internal conversation.

"Mukta, the most important task starts now. We have to control the bleeding quickly and precisely if we are to save the mother."

I tried to peer over the shoulder of my senior. Through the small incision I saw only a pool of blood. How was he going to find the incision in the uterus and suture it? Will the suture be strong enough to hold the friable tissues? Will it control the bleeding? It was truly a work of art, practice, and confidence as the surgeon took the first stitch and tightened the knots with precision. This stitch would serve as the anchor for the life-saving thread that would close the incision made on the uterus to deliver the baby.

The suture thread was an absorbable one, as it was inside the body. At this time in the 1980s we used natural material called catgut suture, made from cat or sheep dried intestine. Literally, one life to save another! The circle of life.

The miracle of childbirth is difficult to describe. Being a witness evokes such a feeling of gratitude indeed. I saw many mothers endure intense pain coupled with tremendous physical trauma, a tearing of the tissues to bring life into the world. I have used the needle and thread to suture the accidental tears or the intentional cut made in the pelvic floor to ease the baby's passage. As I would repair the tears, I often was amazed at how oblivious the mothers were to my presence. The joy of celebrating their new life was their focus.

Different layers of tissue require different types of stitches. I had practiced many times on plastic models, but the real thing was different—the act felt sacred. The thread was my instrument to heal the wounds that were needed to bring life! During my time as an OBGYN resident, I used the needle and thread many times.

## The Last Stitch

The last stitch is just as important.

First you have to make sure all the other stitches are still in place. You check that the line of alignment is absolutely as desired. You make sure there is no bleeding from the other stitches. You make sure you've done all you need to do before you close and tie off. To undo that last stitch could cause more damage. You see, there's a lot of tension. How much tautness and pressure do you put on that final stitch? You want it to be firm. You want it to hold everything with confidence, but at the same time, be gentle enough that it doesn't cut through the tissue. If the stitch is too tight, it can necrose the tissue because its blood supply needs to be maintained and adequate. Thus, you hold the paradoxes of firm, secure, and gentle again.

Before you tell the nurse to cut the thread, you must decide how much of that length you want to keep so that it doesn't unravel, heals properly, and the thread doesn't protrude or irritate the surrounding tissue. Keeping all that in mind, you decide what kind of stitch to take. Then you indicate to the nurse where you want the stitch cut. When you are done, you take a piece of gauze and you wipe it over and make sure the incision is secure, that there is no oozing or gaping. Then you examine your piece of artwork. You either smile, or you see there's an area of concern. If so, do you need to take another stitch elsewhere or not? Finally, you look for approval from the other people who are assisting you. Because it is teamwork.

The first and the last stich are so important. They each lay the foundation for the interior healing for the rest of the life. Then I say a prayer that the person's body will not reject it but has the strength and immunity to heal.

## Life is Reflection

There is something powerful about the image of stitches and scars deep inside a person's body, especially inside a mother, anyone who is struggling to thrive in the midst of complexity. Our physical wounds, our emotional scars, are often invisible. Technology may permit imaging of every layer of our bodies, but technology cannot show soul-level healing. Some places cannot be reached with a mirror. But with the mirror of reflection we can weave together the stitches and threads of our lives into a meaningful tapestry.

We never name it as such, but our whole life is reflection.

I always got my children to write book reports. It's such a joke in our home, now. Every time they read a book, I would read the same book, too, and we each wrote a book report. They had to summarize the book in a few paragraphs so that we could get the essence of that book. Sometimes I had them write personal essays. My children now thank me for those projects and share with gratitude about how important it was for them, but it was such a chore in our house back then.

That's all coming from reflecting, but we never called it reflecting.

THERE'S a lot of talk today about "medical narrative" as if the idea were new. But what do we do in medicine? We ask the patient to reflect on what brought them to the hospital and tell us. Then we reflect back on the knowledge we've gained over years, reflecting on similar patients we've seen. We go back to our memories in our brain and come up with a differential diagnosis. Reflection is such a part of who we are as humans.

When something comes naturally to us, we discount its value, saying "Oh, that's just what I do." It is by naming reflection that we can be intentional about it. Inviting conscious reflection can improve our practice of medicine.

What if reflecting were part of your day-to-day existence? But "reflecting on the fly" takes practice. Each little nugget of reflection can become deeply ingrained and something you can draw on later as needed. Events will have different meanings at different times in your life. These stories happened throughout my life, but I didn't reflect on many of them until this recent season of my life.

I'm called to voice out loudly that we all need to be there for each other, giving permission to show up authentically and share the stories of our lives. Happy and hard stories. My own stories come from reflection, some drawn out of me in a caring, courageous process of reflection, sometimes in solitude with myself, more often in trustworthy conversation with others.

I keep asking myself, "How can I continue to role model by sharing my own authentic reflections and being present for the reflection of others?" It is important to offer empathetic listening, which creates a safe space that makes someone feel brave to share their stories. This leads to a sense of community and belonging. And that helps people overcome isolation, which is one root cause of burnout.

## My Three Questions, Revisited

*Who am I? Where do I belong? How do I heal as I strive to serve?*
The way I accept and embrace other people flows from my
answers to these essential questions.

My life principle acknowledges that who I am is an interde-
pendence with God *and* with the people in my life. I say, "Dear
God, I don't know how to do this" or "I cannot do it by myself."
Initially expressed as prayer, I experience the people in my life
as answers to my prayers and as gifts from God.

Intertwining and guiding my life values is the universal
principle of *wholeness,* which I practice through searching,
acceptance, trust, and surrender. Although I wear many hats
and carry out multiple roles on a daily basis, each is fulfilled
from this deep, interrelated core.

I know we do not have a choice *if* we will leave a legacy, but
we can be mindful of *what* we want the legacy to be. I am still
searching.

Recently I heard from a coworker. She said she had been
speaking to a staff person I worked with since my training days
in 1995 through my varied roles as a resident in training, as a
faculty, as clinic director, associate program director, and then
even more closely as chair of the department of medicine. She
told my coworker that she had seen me in all these roles, but I
was the same Mukta, I had not changed. I hope this doesn't
sound boastful to mention. Her comment meant a lot to me
because it affirms that I'm walking my talk. I have answered
"Who am I?" with "I am myself."

While I continue to search for the legacy I hope to leave, I
want to continue doing my best, being intentionally kind and
grateful, and using the gifts I am blessed with to help all I can
and strive to leave the world a little better.

As I search, I stand with feet that are grounded in faith,

trust, and courage and with eyes that look up to the light for continued guidance.

—

*Your right is to work only, but never to the fruits thereof. Let not the fruit of action be your object, nor let your attachment be to inaction.*

BHAGAVAD GITA

THE END

# ACKNOWLEDGMENTS

*Building community is to the collective as spiritual practice is to the individual.*

GRACE LEE BOGGS

I am blessed that the medical team I work with includes some medical professionals who understand our shared covenant. Each of us knows that we are here to do our work together and that we are each important to the task at hand. The community we've created is one of people and place. Many thanks to the University of Tennessee Health Science Center College of Medicine and its Chattanooga campus which provided me a container of belonging in which I've grown in my profession and as a person. I also give thanks to the cities of Dayton and Chattanooga for the community of belonging I found and for being home as my children grew up.

I owe a deep gratitude to my parents, Shyam and Shashi Parashar, now retired physicians, for teaching me by example to be a vocational partner in medicine. They also showed me how to be a wholehearted citizen of the world, connecting to people from all walks of life.

I am especially grateful to my wonderful friends that have made this book possible. Indrani, thank you for sharing your amazing gift and talent for seeing and capturing what is only understood by the soul. You have been inspiring me since we were twelve! I remain forever grateful to Yvonne for her gentle nudging over brunch on New Year's Day 2016, inviting me to put my stories in a book. Our journey began at the hospital in 2001 during my team's investigative work with her husband, Rob. Our connection from the outset was at a deeper level, our spirits connected. The friendship has continued over the years, and I draw strength from her steadfast faith, courage, and ability to find grace and mercy in every event. Over the years she has not only heard my stories, but heard my soul, read my eyes, felt my emotions, and selflessly consented to help shape the first manuscript with authentic grace and literary elegance. If it had not been for her gentle invitation, this book would not be possible. Namaste!

I feel fortunate to know Shelly Francis, who has been my friend since we first met at a Center for Courage & Renewal retreat in 2012. We bonded over cute but comfortable shoes, joking about the metaphor of walking your talk in your favorite shoes. She interviewed me for the Center's book, *The Courage Way*, which she authored, including my story in the chapter on self-care. I am grateful she said yes when I asked her to help me publish this book. Shelly created a joyful and safe space to expand the depth of my stories relating my passion for physician well-being. It feels like we have a soul agreement to bring this book to fruition.

I am truly grateful to Erin S. Lane for her expertise and experience in preparing me for becoming a visible author and accompanying me through the book launch. I am deeply grateful for Herdley Paolini, Hanna Sherman, and Penny

Williamson for their friendship and thought partnership, not only during this book's creation but for many years as fellow facilitators with the Center for Courage & Renewal.

I thank Scott Ward for allowing me to include his story and poem in chapter 20, Match Day. For all the people who have shared their time and presence with me, I would like to lift up my entire community of family, friends, students, residents, patients, and their families. I've known so many patients whose stories I didn't share here, but our relationships and what I've learned by knowing them have been meaningful.

Above all, I am grateful to my parents and children for their love, support and trust. Parenting does not come with guidelines as do many medical treatments! Thus, my parenting was one of trial and learning from error with much prayer and faith. My children continue to love me in spite of my shortcomings. My children are gifts that keep on giving: Natasha and her husband, Rajas, and Nikhil and his wife, Anuja. They have given me the invitation—and more importantly, the permission —to be me, to be myself with no pretenses in whichever hat I wear. They have shown me how to be my own best friend and to belong, a gift I am truly grateful for!

To you, the reader, thank you for allowing me to share my journey, one blessed by so many who have touched my life.

—

*Gratitude unlocks the fullness of life. It turns what we have into enough, and more. It turns denial into acceptance, chaos to order, confusion to clarity. It can turn a meal into a feast, a house into a home, a stranger into a friend. Gratitude makes sense of our past, brings peace for today and creates a vision for tomorrow.*

MELODY BEATTIE

# NOTES

## Introduction

1. Christopher J. L. Cunningham, Ph.D., Mukta Panda, Jeremy Lambert, Greg Daniel, and Kathleen DeMars, "Perceptions of Chaplains' value and impact within hospital care teams," *J Relig Health.* Aug 2017: 10.1007/s10943-017.
2. Rainer Maria Rilke, *Letters to a Young Poet*, trans. M. D. Herter (New York: Norton, 1993), 35.
3. William Stafford, "The Way It Is," in *The Way It Is: New and Selected Poems* (Minneapolis: Graywolf Press, 1998), 24.
4. Terry Tempest Williams, *When Women Were Birds: Fifty-four Variations on Voice* (New York: Picador, 2012), 228.

## 3. Connecting the Dots

1. U.S. Citizenship and Immigration Services. Conrad 30 Waiver Program, https://www.uscis.gov/working-united-states/students-and-exchange-visitors/conrad-30-waiver-program.

## 7. Differences and Discrimination

1. Saeid B. Amini, "Discrimination of International Medical Graduate Physicians by Managed Care Organizations: Impact, Law and Remedy," 2 *DePaul J. Health Care L.* 461 (1999).
2. Ahmad Masri, M.D. and Mourad H. Senussi, M.D., "Trump's Executive Order on Immigration--Detrimental Effects on Medical Training and Health Care," *N Engl J Med* 2017;376:e39 doi:10.1056/NEJMp1701251,
3. Aba Osseo-Asare, MD1; Lilanthi Balasuriya, MD2; Stephen J. Huot, MD, PhD1; et al. "Minority Resident Physicians' Views on the Role of Race/Ethnicity in Their Training Experiences in the Workplace." *JAMA Netw Open.* 2018;1(5):e182723 doi:10.1001/jamanetworkopen.2018.2723.

## 8. House Calls

1. Nikhil Panda, "Dear Intern," *RAS E-News*, July 2019, Resident and Associate Society, American College of Surgeons, https://www.fac-s.org/publications/newsletters/ras-news/july-2019/dear-intern-letters.

## 9. Walking in a Patient's Shoes

1. *The Internal Medicine Milestone Project*, A Joint Initiative of The Accreditation Council for Graduate Medical Education and The American Board of Internal Medicine (2015), https://www.acgme.org/Portals/0/PDFs/Milestones/InternalMedicineMilestones.pdf.
2. Leo Eisenstein, "To Fight Burnout, Organize," *N Engl J Med* 2018; 379:509-511 doi: 10.1056/NEJMp180377.

## 10. Face to Face

1. Stacey Chang, M.S., and Thomas H. Lee, M.D. "Beyond Evidence-Based Medicine," *N Engl J Med* 2018; 379:1983-1985 doi: 10.1056/NEJMp1806984.

## 12. Turning Points

1. Nicole M. Cranley, Christopher J.L. Cunningham and Mukta Panda (2015): "Understanding time use, stress and recovery practices among early career physicians: an exploratory study," *Psychology, Health & Medicine*, 2016;21(3):362-7. doi: 10.1080/13548506.2015.1061675. Epub 2015 Jul 6.

## 16. The Good Physician

1. Two well-being initiatives in particular arose from this mandate: "Improving Physician Well-Being, Restoring Meaning in Medicine," Accreditation Council for Graduate Medical Education, https://acgme.org/What-We-Do/Initiatives/Physician-Well-Being and the Action Collaborative on Clinician Well-Being and Resilience launched in 2017 by the National Academy of Medicine as a network of more than 60 organizations committed to reversing trends in clinician burnout, https://nam.edu/initiatives/clinician-resilience-and-well-being/.
2. Greg Feldman Memorial, http://www.gregfeldmanmemorial.org.
3. Donald M. Berwick, Thomas W Nolan, and John Whittington, "The Triple Aim: Care, Health, and Cost," *Health Affairs*, 2008 27:3, 759-769.

4. Thomas Bodenheimer and Christine Sinsky, "From Triple to Quadruple Aim: Care of the Patient Requires Care of the Provider," *Annals of Family Medicine,* vol. 12,6 (2014): 573-6. doi:10.1370/afm.1713.

5. Rishi Sikka, Julianne M. Morath, and Lucian Leape, "The Quadruple Aim: care, health, cost and meaning in work," *BMJ Quality & Safety,* Oct 2015, 24 (10) 608-610; doi:10.1136/bmjqs-2015-004160.

6. Accreditation Council for Graduation Medical Education, CLER Evaluation Committee, *CLER Pathways to Excellence: Expectations for an Optimal Clinical Learning Environment to Achieve Safe and High Quality Patient Care, Version 1.1,* (Chicago: 2017), 30.

7. "Promoting Physician Well-Being and Engagement," online resources, programs, policy and research results for the University of Tennessee College of Medicine Chattanooga Campus and its Graduate Medical Education (GME) Programs, http://www.comchattanooga.uthsc.edu/subpage.php?pageId=1419.

8. Adam B. Hill, M.D., "Breaking the Stigma—A Physician's Perspective on Self-Care and Recovery," *N Engl J Med* 2017; 376:1103-1105 doi: 10.1056/NEJMp1615974.

9. "14th Dalai Lama to visit Madison for live-streamed event on global well-being," Center for Healthy Minds, University of Wisconsin—Madison, https://centerhealthyminds.org/news/14th-dalai-lama-to-visit-madison-for-live-streamed-event-on-global-well-being, and "The World We Make: Well-Being 2030," recorded video, March 9, 2016, https://centerhealthyminds.org/the-world-we-make.

## 17. A How to Live Curriculum

1. Salvatore Mangione, MD and Marc J. Kahn, MD, MBA, MACP, "The old humanities and the new science at 100: Osler's enduring message," *Cleveland Clinic Journal of Medicine,* Vol 86 Number 4, April 2019, 233.

2. *Learn the Eight Dimensions of Wellness* (poster), US Substance Abuse and Mental Health Administration (SAMSA), https://www.store.samhsa.gov/product/Learn-the-Eight-Dimensions-of-Wellness-Poster-/SMA16-4953.

3. Vivek Murthy, "Work and the loneliness epidemic: Reducing isolation at work is good for business," *Harvard Business Review,* September 2017, https://hbr.org/coverstory/2017/09/work-and-the-loneliness-epidemic.

4. Sara Berg, "Family doctors spend 86 minutes of 'pajama time' with EHRs nightly," American Medical Association, (September 11, 2017), https://www.ama-assn.org/practice-management/digital/family-doctors-spend-86-minutes-pajama-time-ehrs-nightly.

## 19. What Am I Fighting For?

1. Barbara Oakley, Areil Knafo, Guruprasad Madhavan, and David Sloan Wilson (eds.), *Pathological Altruism*, Oxford University Press, (New York: 2012).

## 20. Match Day

1. David Whelan, "Alvin Roth Receives Economics Nobel For Flawed Residency Match System," *Forbes*, (October 15, 2012), https://www.forbes.com/sites/davidwhelan/2012/10/15/alvin-roth-receives-economics-nobel-for-flawed-residency-match-system/#c3ee60c376c9.
2. Campus CARES and CARE Teams at the University of Tennessee are based on the NaBITA (National Behavioral Intervention Team Association) model, a nationally recognized authority for Behavioral Intervention Teams. See http://uthsc.edu/care-team.
3. Ramin Walter Parsa-Parsi, MD, MPH, "The Revised Declaration of Geneva: A Modern-Day Physician's Pledge," *JAMA*, 2017;318(20):1971-1972 doi:10.1001/jama.2017.16230.

# ABOUT THE AUTHOR

**Mukta Panda, MD, MACP, FRCP–London,** is an award-winning physician, speaker, and facilitator whose work seeks to transform the heart of patient care and medical education. Dr. Panda is the Assistant Dean for Well-Being and Medical Student Education and a Professor of Medicine at the University of Tennessee College of Medicine at Chattanooga and is former chair of the Department of Internal Medicine. Author of over 60 publications, her writing focuses on educational and curricular development, spirituality in medicine, addressing fatigue and stress, and promoting the well-being of health care professionals.

Dr. Panda grew up in India and has studied, trained, and practiced medicine in India, London, and Saudi Arabia before pursuing another residency training and practice in the US. She is a Fellow of the Royal College of Physicians (RCP–London) and a Master in the American College of Physicians (ACP). The daughter of two physician/educators, she is the proud mother and mother-in-law of Natasha and Rajas, and Nikhil and Anuja.

She is an active member of the Collaborative for Healing and Renewal in Medicine (CHARM), a national working group to promote resident physician well-being and decrease job burnout. Locally, she co-chairs the Physician Well-Being Task Force and serves on the board of directors for the Chattanooga-Hamilton County Medical Society and the Center for Mindful Living.

Dr. Panda has received many awards and recognitions, including the Parker J. Palmer Courage to Teach Award from the Accreditation Council for Graduate Medical Education (ACGME) in 2008. Mukta received the 2016 ACP Award for Outstanding Educator of Residents and Fellows. In 2012 Dr. Panda accepted the Mahatma Gandhi Pravasi Gold Medal honor at the House of Lords in London. The Tennessee Chapter of ACP recognized her with the Laureate Award in 2011. She also received the Tennessee Medical Association Distinguished Service Award in 2018 for her work on the issue of physician well-being.

She co-founded LifeBridge, a physician vitality and well-being initiative of the Chattanooga-Hamilton County Medical Society. She leads the University of Tennessee Health Science Center (UTHSC) Chattanooga chapter of Women in Medicine and Science (WIMS) and founded the UTHSC College of Medicine chapter of the Gold Humanism Honor Society.

Dr. Panda is dedicated to creating healthier lives for the medical students and residents she is leading and her colleagues, not only for their own wholeness and well-being, but also because she knows this is crucial to a healthy workplace and better patient outcomes. To rejuvenate, Mukta likes to take long walks, cook good Indian meals, and plan surprise parties for her loved ones.

**Author's note:** Stories about my work as a clinician and educator do not reflect the opinion of the University of Tennessee Health Science Center (UTHSC) College of Medicine, the UTHSC College of Medicine at Chattanooga, or its affiliate hospital. I have changed people's names and certain identifying characteristics, especially where medical histories are described. Where actual names are used, permission was granted.

# EXPLORE YOUR WELL-BEING

Dr. Mukta Panda is available for speaking engagements, workshops, retreats, and organizational consulting. Please visit www.MuktaPandaMD.com for more information.

## ABOUT CREATIVE COURAGE PRESS

**CREATIVE
COURAGE
PRESS**

Creative Courage Press, LLC, is a brand-new independent publishing company founded in 2020 by Shelly L. Francis, inspired by the people she met while writing *The Courage Way: Leading and Living with Integrity*. Now, in collaboration with others authors, we are creating courage for the complexity of being human.

Get to know the essential voices of our remarkable authors and their refreshing ideas for leading change from the heart. Together we hope to generate meaningful conversations in our communities.

Visit us online to get fortified with resources and reflections for creating your own courageous way of life. As we grow, we invite you to grow with us.

www.CreativeCouragePress.com
hello@CreativeCouragePress.com